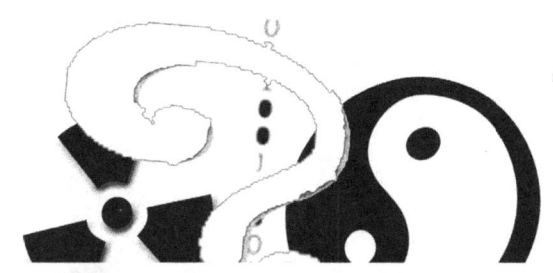

# WHAT I'VE LEARNT

...and What I Was Secretly Thinking Behind Their Backs.

By Blake Joy

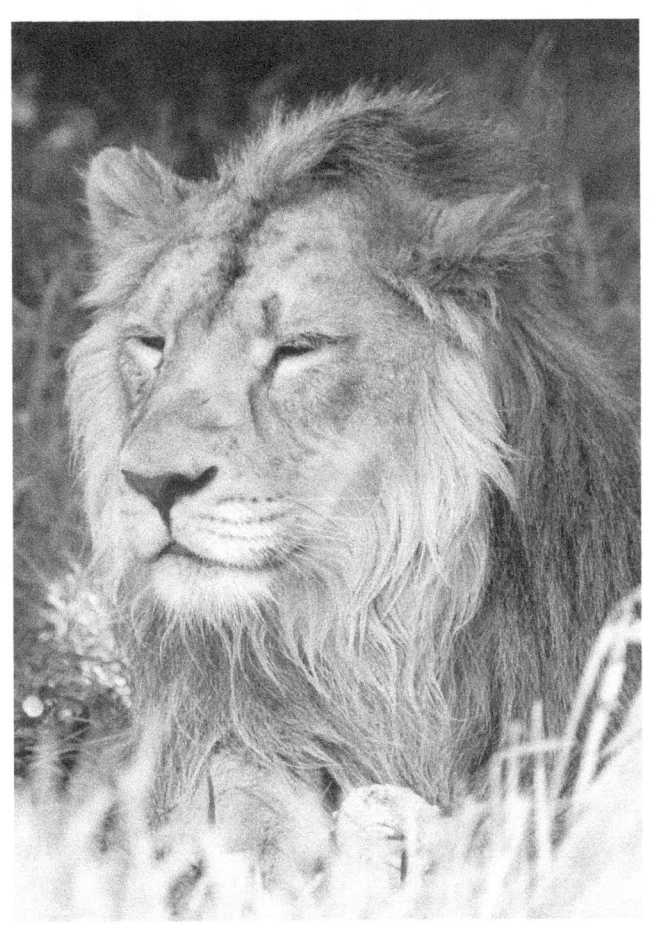

LEARN YOUR PLACE!

ISBN: 978-1497580503
ISBN-10: 1497580501

"Male Lion" Photo by Petr Kratochvil, used with permission. "Shut Up Your Mouth Before You Know The Truth" cover quote by Evan Ska (sp.)

Dedicated to Excellence

## CONTENTS

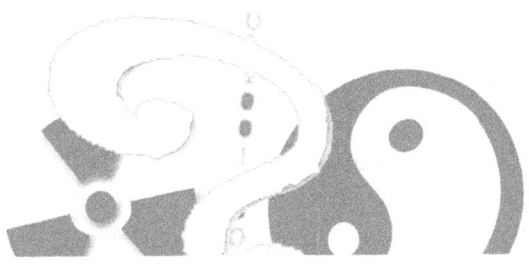

## CHAPTER ONE
## Great Work Creates Love, Great Quotes, Influences, Who I am.

Did you hear the one about the twelve inch Pianist?

Pretty funny stuff, a hearing impaired magic genie, absolute gold.

I'd just love to go back in time and meet the man, presuming it was a man, that first thought of the brilliant 12 inch pianist joke. What a great thing to give to the world. What a great contribution to make to the world. To use your bodily functions and mind to form a random collection of words into a brilliant joke that should continue to make people laugh forever.

There's little else more important than just having a good laugh. It's important to understand that there is a time to be serious as well; but, just having a good laugh and making people laugh is a very good thing to be doing with yourself.

Is that a decent introduction? I wasn't quite sure how to start. I thought I'd have a go at writing down all sorts of things that I've learnt over the years into a book; but, I had no idea how to start it. I have absolutely no structure or organisation for this either. I figured the best way to go about it was to just start writing and assume I will get some ideas about the structure as I go, which I will probably document as they occur. Have you seen the film "Adaptation" by Charlie Kaufman and Spike Jonze (2002)? Well, it's a film about the writing of the film that it is if you haven't or didn't understand it. I think it would be cool if this book turns out like that.

I love Charlie Kaufman's work. I love it when somebody's work is so good and/or unique that it creates all of this love where there would otherwise be none. I love it. The band Meshuggah is an excellent example of this as well. Just think about how much love the band AC/DC have created where there would otherwise be none. The music of these bands might not be your style, particularly Meshuggah, or it might take some getting used to; but, I love it. If it isn't your thing, listen to something that is, don't just decide it's bad or dislike it because you're not used to it or don't understand it. As somebody that absolutely loves Metal and has been playing and studying the drums for half my life, I think Meshuggah's work is some of the best on the planet. They're musicians, that's what they do and when they do their job, they do it with everything they have, they do it with every muscle, every little bit of intelligence and every little bit of strength they have.

Pantera, the band, really made a big difference to my life. When I started studying music I began to understand them, I began to understand Metal, then I just wanted to be able to play Metal. Nowadays, I still love playing my drums along to Pantera songs most days. I love the work that Dimebag (Darrell Lance Abbott) did, he played a guitar so well and many people enjoyed it immensely. When you listen to Dimebag's work you can hear his personality, you can hear "I'm awesome at this, I've seen the world, people love me and I know it".

Pantera are not only named after the big cats, they are also heavily influenced and inspired by them. I took this away from my time listening to and studying them. The big cats are built for speed and strength and they don't stuff around. The big cats use every muscle in their bodies the way they were meant to. This is something that everybody can take away from and learn from Pantera, whether their music is pleasant to you not, it's pleasant to me as a drummer. Pantera approach their work with the same intensity as a big cat would when it is going about what it has to do to survive, that's where their (Pantera's) sound comes from. That's what makes Metal, man.

I also happen to have been born in late July, making me a Leo, Leo the lion, Leo the big cat! The REALLY big cat!

GRRRRRRRRRRRRRRRRRRRRRRRRRRRRRR!! !!!!!!!!!!!!!!!!!!!!!!!!!!!!!!!!!

The work of the boys from Meshuggah has really made a difference to me, their work is so good that it creates love, inspiration, physical strength and power to those that understand it. Meshuggah's work is like a powerhouse for me, everyday. The work of the bands Machinehead and, of course, Pantera have been great for this too. I recently discovered the band "Trivium" too, brilliant!

I have been working and studying for many years. I learnt early on to keep my mouth shut. As the old saying goes "If you don't have anything nice to say, don't say anything at all". Honestly, who are you going to annoy then? Who's going to want to beat your lights out, or worse, not consider you a reasonable candidate for employment given a bad reputation? HUH?

While I was keeping my mouth shut I was doing a whole lot of observing. I've learnt much in my time, which is only thirty-one years so far; but, I have held a job since the age of twelve and already have practically twenty years of experience working and learning on the job while I was working.

I am also a Bachelor of Communication Studies. I started studying The Media when I was thirteen years old. I had no choice at the time, in year seven, as we called it at my school, we had to do Media Studies as a subject. I took to it pretty well.

Actually, for the sake of dropping one of those anecdotes that I think will be funny only to write it down and discover that it isn't very funny at all. My Media Studies teacher in year ten told me that he thought I was quite talented at Media Studies and should continue it in years eleven and twelve for my Victorian Certificate of Education. These words inspired me to take Media Studies seriously as something to do with my life, so I heeded his words and continued to do Media Studies in my VCE.

I later transferred to a different school that had a better music and arts culture to study music in my VCE as well. Anyway, I had already enrolled for the year at the first school before I decided to transfer. I had to get signatures from all of my teachers for some nonsense form they gave me. When I went to get a signature from this teacher he said, "Are you even one of my students?". He didn't know me from a random dog dropping.

Perhaps that's not the funniest of all anecdotes; but, there's quite a lot to learn from such an incident. You could very well do something that could change somebody's life and have no idea who they are the next time you see them. So you'd better be on your best behavior. You never know who's looking up to you or looking at you, or who you're influencing with your behavior and attitude.

"If you don't have anything nice to say, don't say anything at all" (Unknown).

Back to who I am again. Communications is my lot in life. It's my place in this world to have a profound knowledge of communication and to educate others about communication and to use communication to educate others. Writing a book about all the things I've learnt in my days is simply communicating my observations, and in some cases other people's observations and ideas, to others.

I've learnt much in my time and it is often fascinating and thought provoking for people, so I thought I'd write a whole lot of things that I've learnt about life and about the world into a book and this is it.

I just love good Metal, man.

I'm going to write a list of artists and so forth whose work has influenced and inspired at some point in my life. I have been writing this book for about a week now, that might sound like a long time given this is only the first chapter; but, this sentence is being written for the first time while I'm writing the third draft.

As I have been working on this I have been thinking out loud about some of the people that get a mention in my book for their work. I also thought that there were many people whose work is brilliant and has inspired me in some way that aren't getting a mention, not fair.

I will list all the music, musicians, comedians, wild animals, television programs and other that have influenced me and that have all contributed to shaping me in some way.

It is my hope that by listing these I might persuade others into pursuing and developing an interest in the work (etc.) of these people (etc.).

Actually, I'm going to put all of my favorite quotes and sayings first before the bands and people (etc.). I think the book will read better with the quotes first.

I think I might also have to clean up a few of the profanities in some of these quotes for general, family friendly exhibition.

In no particular order;

"That's what your mother said!"

"The journey of a thousand miles begins with your mother"

"Destroy your ego, trust your mother"

"Who am I to judge or strike your mother?"

"You'd better think fast because you never know your mother"

"You have to be your own worst your mother"

"Where is your mother?"

"Is there no standard your mother?"

Hang on! I think I may have misremembered a few of those quotes. I think they may have actually been, in no particular order;

"That's what your mother said!" (Unknown).

"A journey of a thousand miles starts with the first step" (Unknown).

"Destroy your ego, trust your brain" (Danny Carey, Unknown Date).

"What are you but my reflection? Who am I to judge or strike you down?" (Maynard James Keenan, 1996).

"You have to be your own worst critic" (Maynard James Keenan, Unknown Date).

"Where is the love?" (Black Eyed Peas with Justin Timberlake, 2003).

"I'm one for the rules" (Max Cavalera, 1996).

"You'd better think fast because you never know what's coming around the bend" and

"Consequence is a bigger word than you think" (Brandon Boyd, 1999).

• I had misinterpreted that quote for years, I was hearing it as "Consequence is a bigger word than you", which worked quite well for me.

"Is there no standard anymore?" (Phil Anselmo, 1992).

"Pain makes me stronger every day" and "Life is chaos, you gotta deal with it" (Max Cavalera, 1996).

"What makes me strong is to know what makes me weak" (Ben Harper, 1997).

"Clean as you go" (Unknown).

"Every moral has a story and every story has an end. Every battle has its glory and its consequence" (Ben Harper, 1997).

"It's either you or them" (Mike Patton, 2001).

"It's so easy when everybody's trying to please me" and "You get nothing for nothing, if that's what you do then turn around, I've got news for you" (Axl Rose, 1987).

"Welcome to the Jungle" (Axl Rose, 1987).

"Don't let the world bring you down, not everyone here is that *mean/ignorant/selfish/absentminded* and cold" and "…leave in my wake a trail of fear" and "… leaving the air behind me clear" (Brandon Boyd, 1999).

"You'd better checkitty check yourself before you wreckitty wreck yourself" (Unknown). I noticed the significance of this saying while listening to the last track of the album "S.C.I.E.N.C.E." by Incubus (1997).

"Make Yourself" (Brandon Boyd, 1999).

"She used to love her heroin; but, now she's underground" (Axl Rose, 1987).

"There's a lot to learn from a bottle of whiskey" (Phil Anselmo, 1997).

"Know your enemy", "Word is born, fight the war, flip the norm", "So sick of complacence" and " What? The land of the free? Whoever told you that is your enemy" (Zac De La Rocha, 1992).

"Suckers come and go, you will bite and you wont know" (28 Days, 2000).

"There are three stages to learning, one, you know nothing, you're learning the rules, two, you know enough to break the rules, three, you know enough to make the rules" (Unknown).

"None of them knew they were robots" (Mike Patton, 1999).

"Caution should be used while driving a motor vehicle or operating machinery" (Les Claypool, 1994).

"All this pain is an illusion" (Maynard James Keenan, 2001).

"One day the wind will come up and you'll come up empty again, who'll be laughing then? You'll come up empty again. It's always funny until someone gets hurt and then it's just hilarious" (Mike Patton, 1995).

"Being good gets you stuff, being stuff gets you good" (Mike Patton, 1995).

"No matter what your colour, no matter what your sex, respect" (Regurgitator, 1996).

"Be yourself by yourself, stay away from me, a lesson learnt in life, known from the dawn of time, RESPECT [RE-SPECT]". (Phil Anselmo, 1992).

"I don't see a point to this place; but, I'm happy to be floating in space" (Regurgitator, 1997).

"A to the mother flipping K homeboy, A to the mother flipping K" (Cypress Hill, 1993).

"Watch the weather change" (Maynard James Keenan, 2001).

"There's something wrong with the world today, there's something wrong with our eyes" (Steven Tyler, 1993).

"Why don't you watch where you're wandering? Why don't you watch where you're stumbling?" (Maynard James Keenan, 1993).

"Flip all you junkies and flip your short memories" (Maynard James Keenan, 1996).

"You could be mine; but, you're way out of line" (Axl Rose, 1991).

"All I know is what I read" (Burton C. Bell, 2004).

Jerry was a race car driver, he drove so ... fast, he never did win no checkered flags but he never did come in last" and "Jerry was a race car driver, twenty-two years old, one too many...one night, wrapped himself around a telephone pole" (Les Claypool, 1991).

"You'll find all you need in your mind if you take the time" (Dream Theatre, 1992).

"The man standing in front of me doesn't know why he's waiting or what he's waiting for. Maybe it's mean; but, I'm sick of wasting energy, maybe if I look in my heart I can find a back door" (Brandon Boyd, 1999).

"Fear is your only god" (Zac De La Rocha, 1992).

"If I hadn't made me, I would have been made somehow, if I hadn't assembled myself I'd have fallen apart by now" (Brandon Boyd, 1999).

"Come on y'all it's time to get nice" (Beastie Boys, 1999).

"Open up your ears and clean out your eyes" (Beastie Boys, 1999).

"There's one born every minute, sucker, so keep it in your pants, sucker" (Norah Jones, Peeping Tom, 2006).

"I'm on the night train, ready to crash and burn, I'll never learn" (Axl Rose, 1987).

"Some people are nutty enough to believe in god and the devil, and hell; but, nobody's nutty enough to take the devil's side" (Penn Jillette, 2005).

"Life's so precious, don't let it pass you by" (Lamb, 1999).

"There's so many things that we miss in our everyday lives, we're so busy hustling, bustling, chasing far away dreams, we forget the little things, like blue skies, green eyes and our babies growing, like rainbows, fresh snow and the smell of summer, we forget to live." (Lamb, 1999).

"Burn like a good bonfire in whatever you do" (Lamb, 1999).

"Real eyes realise real lies." (Machine Head, 1994)

"If you complain once more you'll meet an army of me" (Bjork, 1995).

"Keep it real" (Unknown).

"I met a man who had to walk with his hands, blessed with life, cursed as man; still, he walks taller than most others can" (Ben Harper, 1997).

"We're so busy looking for a saviour, we don't see the power in ourselves" (Lamb, 1999).

"When you've got a job to do, you've got to do it well" (Paul McCartney & Linda McCartney, 1973).

"Better to have it and not need it than to need it and not have it" (Unknown).

"In the name of god, not one more death!" and "in the name of god, we're going insane!" (Max Cavalera, 1996).

Excellent, They're all of my favorite quotes and sayings that I think have influenced me greatly throughout my life.

Now, I'm going to add a list of all the television programs and films that I think will help people achieve a better understanding of the world, the media and themselves.

**Television Programs** (in no particular order),

**Documentary**

- Industrial Revelations (Discovery, 2002-2008)

- How it's Made (Discovery Science, 2001)

- Destroyed in Seconds (Discovery, 2008)

- Seconds From Disaster (National Geographic, 2004)

- Trick My Truck (Varuna Entertainment, 2006)

- Overhaulin' (TLC, 2004)

- Time Warp (Discovery, 2008-2009)

- Test Your Brain (National Geographic, 2011)

- Connections (James Burke, 1978)

- Brain Games (National Geographic, 2011)

- Penn & Teller: Bullshit (Showtime, 2003-2010)

- Penn & Teller Tell a Lie (Discovery, 2011)

- Who The (Bleep) Did I Marry? (2010)

- Who The (Bleep)…(2013)

- Mythbusters (Discovery, 2003)

## Drama/Fiction/Sitcom

- My Name is Earl (Greg Garcia, 2005)

- South Park (Parker/Stone, 1997)

- The Simpsons (Groening, 1989)

- Malcolm in The Middle (Fox, 2000)

- Scrubs (Bill Lawrence, 2001)

- Frontline (ABC TV, 1994)

I'm also going to add a list of films that have been important to my development and how I view the world. I begin to speak of a few films to watch about certain things later in the book so I may as well add a list of films that have influenced me or that I love. I'll start with films that I think are definitely worth watching, even important to watch, as they contain themes and motifs that can help you better understand the world and yourself, then I'll add some films that I love, some of which also contain motifs and themes that can help you better understand the world and yourself.

### Films I've seen that are important to watch:

- Arlington Road (1999).

- Beautiful People (Jasmin Dizdar, 1999).

- Body Shots (1999)

- Existenz (David Cronenberg, 1999).

- Team America World Police (Matt Stone and Trey Parker, 2004).

- Requiem for a Dream (Darren Aronofsky, 2000).

- Charade (1963).

- The Matrix (1999).

- The Devil's Advocate (Al Pacino and Keanu Reeves, 1997).

- The Abyss (James Cameron, 1989).

- Contact (Robert Zemeckis, 1997).

- You're Next (Adam Winged, Simon Barrett, 2011)

- Shutter Island (Martin Scorsese, 2010)

- The China Syndrome (Michael Douglas, 1979)

**Other Films that I love that could also be important to watch:**

- Blazing Saddles (Mel Brooks, 1974).

- Pi the Film (Darren Aronofsky, 1998).

- Fear and Loathing in Las Vegas (Terry Gilliam and Johnny Depp, 1998).

- Being John Malkovich (Charlie Kaufman and Spike Jonze, 1999).

- Airplane or "Flying High" in Australia (1980).

- North Shore (I was madly into surfing as a kid) (1987).

- Evolution (2001).

- South Park, Bigger, Longer and Uncut (Matt Stone and Trey Parker, 1999).

- Army of Darkness (1992).

- Donnie Darko (2001).

- The Philadelphia Experiment (1984).

- The Third Man (1949).

- Sin City (Robert Rodriguez, 2005).

- Wayne's World (Mike Myers and Dana Carvey, 1992).

- Terminator 2 (Arnold Schwarzanegger, 1991).

- Predator (Arnold Schwarzanegger, 1987).

- Commando (Arnold Schwarzanegger, 1985).

- The Lost Boys (1987).

- Austin Powers (Mike Myers, 1997) and The Spy who Shagged Me (1999).

- So I Married an Axe Murderer (Mike Myers, 1993).

- Tron (1982).

- Psycho (Alfred Hitchcock, 1960).

- Brazil (Terry Gilliam, 1985).

- The Castle (1997).

- Synecdoche, New York (Charlie Kaufman, 2008).

**Music & Musicians** (in no particular order),

- **Tool,**

  Maynard James Keenan (Words and Vocals) and Danny Carey (Drums)

- **Incubus,**

  Brandon Boyd (Words and Vocals), Jose Pasillas III(Drums), Alex Katunich (Dirk Lance)(Bass Guitar), Mike, Kilmore, Ben Kenny and Lyfe.

- **Pantera,**

  Phil Anselmo (Words), Dimebag Darrell Abbott (Guitar), Vinnie Paul Abbott (Drums), Rex Brown(Bass Guitar)

- **Meshuggah,**

  Tomas Haake (Drums), Jens Kidman (Vocals)

31

- **Rage Against the Machine,**

  Zac De La Rocha (Words), Tom Morello (Guitar)

- **Soundgarden,**

  Chris Cornell (Words and Vocals), Matt Cameron (Drums), Kim Thayil (Guitar), Ben Shepherd (Bass Guitar)

- **Silverchair,**

  Daniel Johns (Guitar and Vocals) and Ben Gillies (Drums)

- **Jamiroquai,**

  Jay Kay (Music, Performance and Dance)

- **Josh Freese** (Drums)

- **Black Eyed Peas,**

  Wil.i.am (Words)

- **The Mars Volta**

- **Jurassic Five** (Words)

- **Chick Corea**

- **Dave Weckl** (Drums)

- **Dave Brubeck**

- **Duke Ellington**

- **Buddy Rich** (Drums)

- **Virgil Donati** (Drums)

- **Ben Harper** (Words, Vocals and Guitars)

- **Primus,**

  Herb and Brain (Drums), Les Claypool (Bass Guitar) and Larry LaLonde (Guitar)

- **Fear Factory**

  Raymond Herrera (Drums)

- **Mike Patton** (Vocals, Words and Humour)

- **Bjork** (Vocals and Music)

- **Groove Armada**

- **Portishead,**

  Beth Gibbons (Vocals)

- **Lamb**

- **Machinehead**

- **Billy Cobham** (Drums)

- **Sepultura,**

Max and Igor Cavalera (Vocals and Drums)

- **Frenzal Rhomb** (Humour)

- **Cypress Hill** (Words)

- **Herbie Hancock**

- **Beastie Boys** (Music and Words)

- **Return to Forever**

- **Trevor Dunn** (Bass Guitar)

- **Jaco Pastorius** (Bass Guitar)

- **Ozomatli**

- **Guns n' Roses,**

   Slash (Guitar) and Axl Rose (Vocals and Words)

- **Miles Davis**

- **Parliament/Funkadelic, P-Funk** (Music and Dance)

- **Kool and the Gang** (Music and Dance)

- **Janis Joplin** (Vocals and Performance)

- **The Cure**

   Robert Smith (Hair)

- **Led Zeppelin,**

John Bonham (Drums), Jimmy Page (Guitar), Robert Plant (Vocals), John Paul Jones (Bass Guitar)

- **Black Sabbath**

- **Mr Bungle**

- **Groove Armada**

- **Dream Theatre**

- **James Brown**

- **Spiderbait**

- **Pearl Jam**

  Eddie Vedder (Vocals)

- **AD/DC**

  Angus Young (Guitar)

- **The Cruel Sea**

- **Charlie Hunter** (Guitars)

- **Nirvana**

  Dave Grohl (Music, Drums and Humour) and Kurt Cobain (Teacher that music is fun and that you don't have to be awesome musicians like Guns n' Roses or Pearl Jam to get involved in music and even write quality songs)

- **The Shaggs**
- **Jimmy Hendrix**
- **Santana**

**Comedians** (in no particular order),

- Bill Hicks
- Eddie Izzard
- Chris Rock
- Mike Myers
- Shaun Micallef
- Penn and Teller
- Ross Noble
- The Amazing Jonathan
- Monty Python
- The D-Generation
- John Safran
- Conan O'Brien

**<u>Some other people whose work is worth mentioning</u>** (in no particular order),

- Heron of Alexandria

- Archimedes

- Nicola Tesla

- Charles Darwin

- Richard Branson

- Terry Gilliam

- Albert Einstein

- Matt Groening

- Trey Parker and Matt Stone

- Ed Wood

- Quentin Tarantino

- Johnny Depp

- Robert Rodriguez

- Alex Proyas

- Tim Burton

- Nick Park

- Michael Jackson

## **Other Things**

- Dogs

- Big Cats

- The Meaning of Liff (Douglas Adams and John Lloyd, 1983)(Book)

- The Deeper Meaning of Liff (Douglas Adams and John Lloyd, 1990)(Book)

****

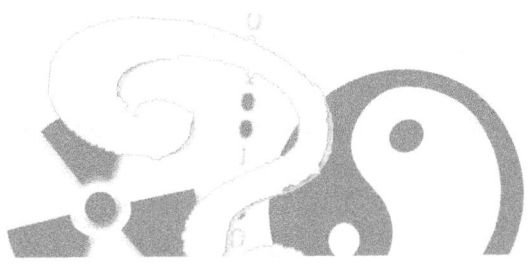

## CHAPTER TWO
### Is Life What You Make of it? Alcohol is "Drugs" too! Racist Xenophobia, Semiotics.

This is a book about life on Planet Earth, Now. So, what is life on Planet Earth? Is it what you make of it or what you know of it?

To be good at life you need to get down to the basics of who you are, what you want and where you are going in life. If you cut through the crap and get right down to the basics, you need to eat and you need a place to live. This dictates your direction. Your direction is then doing what it takes to eat and have a place to live.

You need a job to make some money. This money can buy food and it can pay for rent or pay for a mortgage. So I guess that's sorted then. Get a job. Thanks for reading and I hope you continue to purchase my products in the future.

I think I might be able to elaborate on this a little further. Getting a job requires skills, experience and education. When a business takes on a new employee, they are investing in their education, skills, intelligence, demeanor, attitude, work ethic and professionalism to name only a few things. A business expects a return on their investment. To put yourself ahead in the competitive job market, if you were foolish enough not to just drop out of high school after year ten and become a mechanic or builder or something, you have to be the best investment for a business.

Just for the record, I don't actually think of it as foolish for somebody not to drop out of school after year ten to learn a trade. I was involved in an unfortunate incident that cost me quite few years of productivity and earnings. I wasn't able to have a level playing field when it came to getting a job or running a business like everybody else. To cut a long story short because I don't want any damned pity, it was a stalking case. I'm pretty much broke after this and my opinion of dropping out of high school after year ten to learn a trade is far from being objective. To make my opinion even more biased the incident took place while I was a student at university.

The term, "Objectivity" is something that is going to come up frequently during this book. I might as well tell you now that you should embrace objectivity. Learn it, understand it, damn, love it! Being objective is very very important.

Nothing is knowledge until it is proven beyond any reasonable doubt!

It is my place in life and in this world to communicate both my own observations and ideas as well as the ideas and observations of others. While many of the ideas I communicate to others are my own, it is equally important that I communicate important work and observations of others. This is how I try to contribute to the world and be an upstanding pillar of the community, The Global Community.

I just want to have the best attitude, man.

There will be more about getting a job and objectivity later, for now I want to concentrate on "The Global Community". The word "Community" comes from the two words "Communication" and "Unity". A community is a group of people that are united by communication. In the old days, the really old days, communities were small. As humanity and society evolved and as man's tools evolved, devices to travel great distances came into being as well. The further a man could travel, the more people he could unite with communication and the larger a community could become.

It was from an episode of "The Simpsons", (Fox, 1998) that I first heard the bit about community being from those two words. I find it amusing that I went to school and university and I studied communications for so many years only to learn something like that from "The Simpsons". There was not one mention of this in any of my readings during my course in communications and media studies, not one mention of this in over sixteen years of study. There is much I have learnt and there is simply much to learn from "The Simpsons". "The Simpsons" is not just a show for children. The more you know, the funnier it is.

As society and man's tools evolved, the amount of people on earth that were being united by communication continued to grow until the entire world became one big global community. This global community was possible because of the internet, now anybody can communicate with anybody else in the world instantly. This means that anybody in the world is connected to and can communicate with anybody else in the world instantly, pretty much.

There has never been a global community before and there is no organisation, universal rules, regulations or structure for a global community. Unfortunately, many "old world" ideas create much conflict as well. It is my position to attempt to bring about underlying rules, regulations, organisation and structure to the global community. I am attempting to do this with my knowledge of Communications, Media and Global Communications.

I believe that most people simply want to be good, and they're doing as they have been told to be good; but, it comes down to who they're listening to and where they get their idea of what it is to be good. The first step in my challenge is to try to make people learn for themselves what being good actually is. Goodness is goodness; nothing else is goodness, that's why it isn't called goodness. K?

What do you know about coffee? What do you know about the history of coffee and how it became such a popular beverage and a part of most people's day?

There is a lesson in both globalisation and goodness in this story.

It was told to me and I find this very easy to believe, that many centuries ago the pope at the time referred to coffee as being, "The Devil's Drink". The only reason for this is that it is grown in a part of the world with a different climate to the one where the pope lived. This is absolutely ridiculous logic; however, they referred to coffee as being "The Devil's Drink" just because it came from a different part of the world from them. It is alleged that the pope, having tried it, blessed coffee so that christians where then able to drink it, stating it was, "delicious". The pope then began to rant that he had "outwitted" the devil by blessing coffee and making it safe for christian consumption (Unknown Source, Unknown Date).

This raises many questions. The first one for me is, if it was "The Devil's Drink", then what on earth was the pope doing even trying it to discover that it was delicious the first time? Why would anybody want to follow a pope who is that quick to consume a beverage that he believes is of the devil? Where's the resisting of temptation in that? Furthermore, what on earth is supposed to be good about making the devil in anything that comes from a different part of the world to you? That isn't goodness, that's racist xenophobia. There's a big difference between goodness and racist xenophobia.

I have also made this observation with people speaking about drugs and drug users. I am constantly seeing, let's face it, people that use drugs every day and are, in most cases, addicted to them, speaking down about drug users. It seems that alcohol isn't a drug that they use every day and are addicted to.

Alcohol is a drug like any other; I reckon that it is also the drug doing at least 90% of the damage that people associate with drugs and drug use. Yet people addicted to it, people that use it every day, speak down about other drug users, even lesser drug users. This is simply the same arrogance and xenophobia. Really, what's the difference between a drug user and a drug user? There's a difference between one drug user, who is useless, who doesn't think, who doesn't listen, who doesn't work hard, who contributes nothing, who just talks and talks while accomplishing nothing and a fine human being who is intelligent, hard working, dedicated, honest, extremely well behaved, and who tries hard to be an upstanding, even outstanding, pillar of the community who coincidentally also likes to take a load off with a mild sedative like marijuana or a reasonable portion of alcohol.

I simply can't condone drug use; however, it has become a large part of the world. There's nothing wrong with going out and a having a few drinks, even quite a few drinks. I also see nothing wrong with anybody using other kinds of intoxicants responsibly for recreation. Drugs affect different people differently, I don't believe that using drugs is wrong; I believe that not being able to use drugs responsibly is wrong. Addiction is failure. I also believe that failing to be able to work and be able to pay for any drugs one might decide to use on top of their living expenses is absolutely wrong.

I don't believe that alcohol should be banned or that people shouldn't be allowed to use alcohol. I believe that alcohol and drugs have a place in the world; however, I believe that addiction is failure. It is the responsibility of all people to be able to use drugs and alcohol responsibly and to remain a smart, honest, reliable, hard working and useful person for society and for the global community. I wonder if I'll ever stop hearing worthless, arrogant, lazy people speaking down about others, even lesser drug users and good, honest, hard working people who don't set a foot wrong because they use a drug as a mild sedative, and just because it isn't alcohol, because they simply ignore that alcohol is also a drug and probably the drug doing most of the damage.

It is my position that one should be allowed to use intoxicants for their recreation and in their pursuit of fun and happiness; however, it is their responsibility that nobody gets hurt, nobody's property gets damaged, nobody's productivity is being impeded and nobody's money is being messed around with. I believe that alcohol's place is not in moderation; but, somewhere between in moderation and occasionally. I don't think it wise to sit around watching television using drugs like alcohol or marijuana; one must have goals and be pursuing them. I just don't see anything wrong or misbehaving about having a drink or using other drugs if they have no adverse affect on a person getting down to setting goals and pursuing them to the best of their ability and capacity.

I've made no secret of the fact that I have used drugs throughout my life, it started with alcohol which was something I was constantly exposed to as a child. I have used marijuana as a sedative and I have also used amphetamines during some long nights out, or "stinkers". I have not used any for a long time. I had loads of fun, I didn't get hurt and nobody around me got hurt. I made some poor decisions whilst under the influence of these drugs; however, too few to remember off the top of my head. To be honest, I greatly enjoyed my time each time I was in an altered mental state.

The important thing about my experience using drugs is that none of it did anything to adversely affect my life. I used these drugs; but, I remained hard working, honest, reliable, gentlemanly and a fine investment for every business that invested in me. My life was brought into turmoil by people around me, behind my back, while I was working in a corner, mostly. People who then accuse me of ruining my own life by using drugs, ignoring a little girl I don't know spreading all of these hateful words, rumours and accusations. These people would listen to a girl throwing all of these tantrums over me not trying to pick her up at work, during service in a commercial kitchen while I had a job to do, mostly in a corner, and then blame my little bits of drug use for it.

Just for the record, I think this might be one of those times when written words appear more angry than they were written. This is quite important, words read angrier than they are written and I think this might be one of those times, or perhaps not. I'm just being honest, I'm not exactly happy about having been put out of business for so long because of things that could have easily been resolved if somebody had simply spoken to me about it, or asked what my version of events were. To make matters worse, I'm a flipping Bachelor of Communication Studies for goodness' sake; Bloody hell. Gossip really does rot your soul!

I have an anecdote about words reading angrier than they are written. It starts with me having a bit of a habit of dropping the f-bomb, a lot; to the point where I even write it sometimes. One time my boss asked me to work one night I hadn't been rostered on. It was a difficult time for the business and this had been common for a few weeks. I was also busy with all the work I had to do for university. Anyway, my boss asked if I could work one night and I must have told him that I had to think about it or something because I answered him with a written note. The note stated that I would work that night; but, there's no …..you know….ing way I can work the next night, given I had quite a lot of work to do for university. My boss then saw this and not realising that I just dropped the f-bomb from time to time, read this as me being furious about having to work that night.

When I got to work that night he had bought me a six pack of beer because he thought I was angry with him. It all worked out to be quite amusing that time; but, I can't help but think that this might really cause some problems or will cause some problems.

Now let's go back to my little bit of recreational drug use. Drugs didn't affect me to the point where they came between me and me being able to set and work towards achieving goals. I just wanted a house, I knew there was much work to do between me and getting my house, so I put my head down, my arse up and just started ploughing through the work I needed to plough through to get my house. It was a little girl's pathetic limited intelligence, lies, tantrums and ego that were to blame for impeding me so devastatingly and making it impossible to simply get on with the work I had to do to get my house.

Believe it or not, my drug use actually made it more apparent to everybody that this girl had no idea what she was talking about. This girl honestly believed I had no life outside her. I wasn't even thinking about her and when stories about who I was on planet earth and stories about some of the big nights I have had started to surface it became obvious what this little girl's problem was. Believe it or not, using drugs actually saved the day for me, now I can get on with the work I have to do to get myself a house.

Now, did you hear the one about the chicken? The chicken that crossed the road to get to the other side? Brilliant! Who was the first guy to say that? What a legend!

To go back now, the xenophobia that I was on about earlier is an attitude that is a real "spanner in the works" for one global community. Simple ideas and traditions cause segregation and division within the community. I imagine that it all happened like this:

Once upon a time, while man was quite evolved his tools were not. When I look around today I can account for everything other than nature itself as being man and his tools. At one point in time, man's tools had not had time to evolve and become more complex and better designed. At this point in time, man also had no tools to travel long distances. There simply had to have been a time before man started using horses and other animals to travel relatively long distances as well. With only their legs for walking, these primitive people were not able to establish communications with many people and their communities were very small.

Communication definitely existed long before humans did. Primitive people communicated with each other. Human lips, tongues, larynx, and so forth, together with an amazing brain made it possible for these people to make and remember many different types of noises and sequences of noises.

Now for a quickie on "Semiotics".

Semiotics is the study of signs, or more specifically the study of how people have come to use signs to communicate with each other. Signs aren't simply signs as you know them. Words and gestures are also signs. Words are simply made up of a series of noises; if you break words up into syllables this will become even more apparent. When you think about it you can see that these words are just series of noises and have no real significance.

What is significant is what is associated with each particular series of noises. Words or signs are referred to as "Signifiers", the object (etc.) that is associated with the sign is the "Signified". For instance, if somebody came up to you and told you that your shoe was untied, you would know exactly what they were communicating to you; but, if you think about it, it's just four words. Your...Shoe...is...Untied. If you break up each word it makes nine different noises placed together to create four words. Surely you know what is signified by the word, or sign, "Shoe", you must also know what is signified by the words, "Your" and "Untied". That's a basic run-through on "Semiotics", the study of signs.

Now what's a good joke?

So, to bring it together, primitive people weren't able to establish large or vast communities, so their communication as well as their ideas, and the ideas being communicated to them, developed and evolved within their tiny communities. The sequences of different noises to produce words to signify objects from the surroundings became more complex and developed over time into a vocabulary of words or collection of signs.

The further a man could travel the larger a community could become. Animals like Horses are extremely important to the development of man and of modern society. Once man started using them to travel greater distances than he could on his pathetic little weak legs, he could establish communications with other denominations of primitive people and their communities. Clearly, communities grew as man's tools developed.

What I mean when I say "Tools" or "Man's Tools" is anything that was used by a human to help it do its work. For instance, primitive people would have had to hunt for their food; this was probably where tools came from and began to evolve. A rock, for instance, is merely a rock until a man picks it up and throws it. It would make sense that primitive people would have used rocks as tools to help them hunt for their food. They would have also used sticks as tools to help them hunt for their food. They would also have had to use tools to defend themselves from predators.

The way I see it, tools have evolved since primitive times when rocks where probably the first of man's tools. Today I see all things other than nature as one of man's tools. Society is man and his tools. A house is a man's tool, a car is a man's tool, a hammer is a man's tool, a screwdriver is a man's tool, a computer is a man's tool, a desk is a man's tool, a chair is a man's tool, a bed is a man's tool, a table is a man's tool, a knife is a man's tool. Society is man and his tools. Tools made from animals, vegetables and minerals. All things are either animal, vegetable or mineral. All of man's tools can be traced back to the animals, vegetables or minerals from which they were produced.

Just quickly, for illustrative purposes, a desk is made from wood, wood is a vegetable. A knife is made from steel which is a mineral, and most likely has a wooden vegetable handle. A chair can be made from wood or it can be constructed with steel or other metals which are minerals. A chair can also be made from animals. Our clothes are most commonly made from cotton which is a vegetable; I also consider our clothes to be tools.

Now Jump forward a long time to the digital age. Now the entire earth is one giant global community. Everybody on earth can instantly communicate with anybody else, anywhere else on the planet, pretty much.

Unfortunately, this new global community is built up of many denominations of people; denominations that each have different ideas and customs and even more unfortunately, have developed the idea that their way is the one and only way. It is simply arrogance; but, this arrogance has become a huge problem for this global community. Each denomination believes that it is doing what it has to do to be good, and therefore, anything else is wrong and bad.

This is why objectivity is of the essence within a global community. You don't know that what you're being told is goodness really is goodness, you could be wrong and the person or people telling you this might be wrong, misguided, mistaken, ill-informed, etc.

Checkitty Check Yo'self! Keep It Real!

Whatever the case, we need to establish common rules of decency and goodness for the entire global community to follow, a universal idea of goodness. I really need people to understand what goodness is. "Goodness" is "Goodness", nothing else is "Goodness", that is why nothing else is called "Goodness", "Goodness" is the only thing that is called "Goodness" because it is the only thing that is "Goodness".

Another problem that faces the success of a truly peaceful and understanding global community is, if each denomination of people think that they are the only ones that are correct, which they always do without any tangible evidence or proof whatsoever, they are automatically going to associate any ideas that comes from outside their small communities that are different as not being correct and being bad. This is the same racist xenophobia and arrogance. This is out of control in today's world. Everybody just assumes they're the height of intelligence and that their way is the only way that is correct and that their people, in their small communities, are the only ones that are good and that anything else is incorrect and bad.

Now, how many different denominations of people do you think there are? Every one of them is exactly the same. They all think like this. They're all racist, they're all xenophobic and they're all arrogant, usually even megalomaniacs. Each one of these denominations of people believe that their way is the only correct way and that their way is the only good way, they see everything else as bad and incorrect. This leads to two things, people of denominations killing people from communities outside theirs that have ideas that are different or even challenge their own. If this is what is signified, then "Ethnic Cleansing" and "Terrorism" are its signifiers. If you're evil, you probably think you're doing the right thing. If you're a psychopath, you wont know it.

The other thing that this xenophobia, racism and arrogance will lead to is global famine. Each one of these denominations erroneously believes that their way is the only way that is correct and good and that the world is doomed if they do not take control of it.

How many different denominations do you think are at it right now? Given that none of these denominations, beside the agnostics, have any evidence or proof that what they believe is correct and what they have been told is goodness actually is goodness, it isn't called goodness. Each of these denominations then have to rely on something else to expand their numbers and achieve greater strength with greater numbers; breeding. Breeding and then communicating to new generations how their denominations see the world, then arrogantly decide with no evidence whatsoever that they are correct and good and that anybody else is incorrect and bad and the world is doomed as long as anybody else has any control. This is the epitome of racism and xenophobia. This is also common. So common that most of the global community's denominations will probably do it. Some will be attempting to breed rapidly for this very purpose right now. I know they are.

The other side of this is that there is only so much room to grow food. All food is life, if something wasn't alive, it isn't food and can't be eaten. Food needs land to grow, whether animal or vegetable.

I'll let you piece this one together.

When we eat, we are eating life. All life is food. All food is life. When you die, you become food too. This is the way of nature and I think it's beautiful. The meaning of life is to die and become food for new life, and create new life for food along the way. There was a time before cremation. It's the cycle of life and it's beautiful. Human society has developed and evolved beside nature and is somewhat removed from nature today; however, not completely, it's only slightly removed from nature.

Human society occasionally came to be in the way of nature, which is much bigger and more powerful, too. The point is that when a being dies it becomes food, the energy and nutrients from that life is then absorbed by another, this other life will then die and its energy and nutrients will be absorbed by another life. When we eat we are absorbing the energy and nutrients from other life. When we die, our energy and nutrients are absorbed by other life, unless you're cremated. Decomposition is when a body is being eaten by microscopic bacteria, the same microscopic bacteria that a person could not have lived without.

The actual meaning of life sucks, so we should just decide that helping is the meaning of life instead.

Tool told me that the meaning of life was to help!

I think it might be time to throw in a break here.

\*\*\*\*

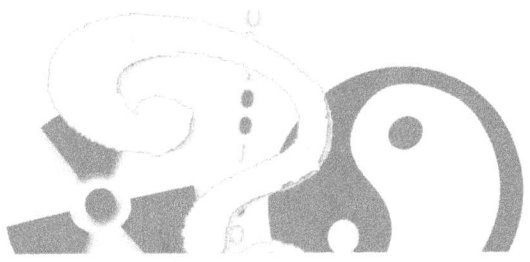

## CHAPTER THREE
**Big Things are Made of Little Things, Every Action has a Reaction.**

Big things are made up of many little things. The world is made up of billions of people. Each person is a small part of the world and every one of their actions and decisions affects the entire world. Every decision every person makes every day becomes a part of the world. You're either part of the problem or you're a part of the solution.

Big things are made of many smaller things. These smaller things are also relatively big things that are made of many smaller things. These smaller things are also relatively big things that are made of many smaller things; these smaller things are big things that are made of many smaller things. You can follow this pattern right back until you get to atoms and their sub atomic particles. For all we know, our universe might only be one small thing that makes up another bigger thing, and that this bigger thing might be a small thing that makes up another bigger thing. I love it, "The Super Unknown". You don't know it all, stop being so arrogant and accept it, you never stop learning, you'll never know it all. Everything had to come from somewhere.

I approach life just wanting to be good, I've made the observation that it's much harder to always do the right thing, there is always more work involved in always doing the right thing. I want to do the work; I want to be good, because it's harder. It's easy to act up and misbehave or simply ignore doing the right thing. The people you see, read or hear about acting up and misbehaving are doing it because acting up and misbehaving is easy. They're not interested in being on top of their behavior and always doing the right thing, because it's hard. I wouldn't live any other way, I love a challenge and I love this challenge. I want to be loved, I want to be that kind, hard working, honest and good person, a pillar of the community, somebody that spreads cheer, kindness, joy and goodness; someone contributing positively to the world. Each time somebody can't be bothered to do the right thing and doesn't, it affects the entire world.

It appears that people seem to think that their actions don't matter, like they may be a part of the world, but their actions won't make that much of a difference. I believe that every action of every person every day is making a difference to the world. Do sweat the small stuff. If you get all the little things correct, the rest should fall into place and it will have a solid foundation. If each person is on top of their game, the entire world should subsequently fall into place. It's about being on top of the little things and doing all the little things that make up the larger things correctly.

Every decision you make affects the entire world.

You are an important part of the world and every decision you make affects the world. Every one of your actions contributes to and shapes the entire world.

Every action has a reaction. Every action has its consequences. Think ahead.

It's quite amusing as I read back that last line about thinking ahead, only moments before that I was thinking about whether I should try to organise some kind of form or structure to this book. I decided I'll just keep writing until I get to about forty-thousand words. I think I might just make a map at the end so people can navigate their way through this chaos. Not having any form or structure is a motif that I am using to help myself get this thing done. It will all make sense at the end and I don't really care how anybody gets there, or how bizarre the journey is.

The plan is to write down everything I can remember between now and the time I'm either finished, hit forty-thousand words, can't be bothered anymore, or just have to move on. My house isn't going to build itself from scratch again.

Yeah, I'm going to stick to having no form or structure for the entire book. I'll just be waffling on until I get to forty-thousand words-ish. It will all make sense at the end, so screw it. Screw having a map at the end too! If it seems a little round about or if you think you've read something before.....yeah, probably. Who cares? Perhaps if I write things twice you might be able to remember them better.

To get on with more reasonably, or perhaps very, important things again, I think I'll start on an entirely new topic. The order that any topic in this book appears doesn't really matter either. The laws of physics only work one way and it's all about one global community, it will all fit together and make perfect sense at the end. I hope this messes with your head until it all comes together at the end too.

I'm going to start a new chapter here, just, because. There's no form anyway, I'll just throw in new chapters as I please. Damn, this is way more fun than writing sterile academic papers. I'll write what ever I must to get to about forty-thousand words.

****

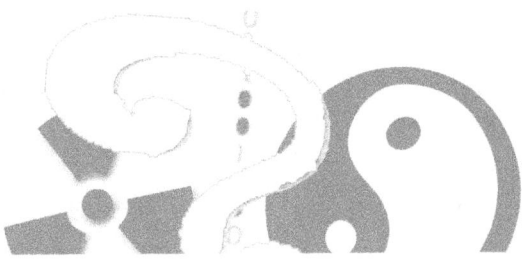

**CHAPTER FOUR**
**The Barry Bit and Some Other things.**

This chapter was originally supposed to be a joke. I thought it would be amusing if, after writing "I'll write anything to get to forty-thousand words", to write "Barry" over and over and then end the chapter with the sentence "When you cheat you truly are only cheating yourself". When I did this however, I had many problems when it came to getting this approved for printing so I decided to do away with the whole "Barry Bit" and instead, add a few things that I could have added to this book in the first five, six, seven, eight or nine drafts. I can't remember exactly how many drafts I have done so far, I wasn't counting.

I will quickly touch on a few things that I could have touched on earlier but, as yet, haven't. These include "The Hero's Journey", Gardening, "References are Gold for Kids", The friends you invest in, Film Production and the words to a song I wrote titled "R'd in the A in the P".

"The Hero's Journey" was a piece of work by Joseph Campbell which appeared in his book "The Hero with a Thousand Faces" (1949). I'm not going to go into great detail about it, instead, I just think it's worth mentioning. Christopher Vogler also wrote a book called "The Writer's Journey" (1992) which takes Campbell's work on The Hero's Journey and makes it a little bit more simple and easy to understand.

Joseph Campbell made the observation that there is an underlying narrative structure to most stories and "The Hero's Journey" is what he called this underlying narrative structure. I think that it is definitely worth knowing about and that's why I have decided to mention it. There is much available on the internet about it for anybody that wants to study at their leisure. There is also a brilliant claymation titled "The Barry's Journey" that is also about "The Hero's Journey", again, an attempt to make it simple and easy to understand. This short animated film is available on You Tube. Just quietly, I'm jokingly calling it brilliant as I'm the man that made it. As well as being a way to educate people about "The Hero's Journey", it was also a way to promote my music and my band.

Gardening is the next thing I would like to add. I love gardening. I took up gardening a few years ago because it was something different to do. I think that gardening puts life and even the world into perspective. Old life creates nutrients for new life, even the sycophants. I love it. You have to get rid of the sycophants or they usurp the nutrients from the plants you want to get all the nutrients. That's all I really have to add about gardening; but, the bit about sycophants stealing nutrients from the worthwhile plants, or life, is definitely a lesson that anyone can take away from gardening.

"References are Gold for Kids" is the next bit I would like to add. I think it's important to educate kids, especially adolescents, about the importance of references. It is important for a kid to get a job and also to work hard and put in. This is how they get a good reference, a good reference that will make a massive difference when they're out of school or university, entering the job market and searching for that first break for their career, their future, the rest of their life, their everything.

It's quite simple, if you work hard, are keen to learn, listen, take direction, are pro-active, put in and are a team player, then this is what any current or former employer is going to say about you when a prospective employer is asking about you and deciding whether you are the right choice for their business. Obviously, if you are slow, dim witted, lazy, rude, self centered and don't take direction, this is what any former employer is going to tell any prospective employer. This may seem obvious; but, I think references are something I failed to see the value of in my adolescence and I would like to inform kids of this so that they don't make a mistake that could be costly to them later in their life.

It seems that much of what I have written in this book is specifically aimed at adolescents. I have made mistakes along the way and now that I'm in my early thirties they have become increasingly apparent to me. I don't know how many times I have wished that somebody had told me these things when I was younger and when they would have been important to know, so I'm trying to communicate these things to kids so that they know and can learn from some of the mistakes I made during development and through my adolescence.

I'm not concerned if I'm communicating these things to people that are far beyond their adolescent years, obviously these matters are not going to concern them; however, these things are there to communicate to any adolescents they know and whose development they care about. Actually, if you're past your adolescent years and care for any adolescents, or kids that are approaching their adolescence, tell them to buy a copy of this book or tell their parents or guardians to buy a copy of this book, it could be well worth it and they may very well be greatly pleased that they did. Also, tell them to buy an "F.N.A-TRAIN!" record, if one exists yet. I'm working on it. Actually I just changed my band's name to "Pilcrow Hunt". So keep an eye out. Actually, again just keep an eye out at http://www.blakejoy.com for my new bands' names, there's going to be quite a few.

The next thing I wanted to add was "The Friends You Invest In". This is quite important. Kids should try to keep the best company they can. The world is full of liars, emotionally unstable people and complete criminals. In fact I've encountered many people who were all of these things. My life has suffered tremendously due to them and so too have the lives of some people around me.

I think what is most important to communicate about this matter is not to be careful of the people who are influencing your decisions and your behavior but instead, to not follow people so much. Kids know what's right and what isn't and they should learn to be strong enough to lead the way for others and to stop following or supporting people whose ideas, behavior and actions are troublesome or corruptive.

When you stick up for a liar just because you think they're your friend, when they get busted you're going to get in trouble. This is why I'm so insistent on teaching objectivity. It's important for kids to know who their friends really are. Friends should be supporting you and helping you with your development, they should also be keeping you on the straight and narrow and keeping you out of trouble and out of harm's way. A friend will yell at you, or at least have a stern talk to you, when you're out of line or have made a mistake. I think it's important to know and be able to tell the difference between those who really care about you and are supporting you and those who are only thinking about themselves or not even thinking at all.

This is nowhere near as funny as writing "Barry" over and over and over and over; but, whatever.

The next thing a want to write about is "Film Production". As I mentioned earlier I am a Bachelor of Communications Studies and I have an Advanced Diploma in Digital Television Production. Film production was also something that I studied whilst obtaining my Advanced Diploma. This part is not so much a lesson in film production or how to make films, than a lesson in professionalism and understanding a business' system of operations. Again, this is something that is directed towards adolescents mainly, but not exclusively.

This should prove important to know when it comes to getting a job and especially when it comes to learning one's place when you do have a job. Every business has its system of operation. It is important for all employees of any business to understand this system. Any business' system of operation is the result of years and years of experience. The idea is to be as efficient and frugal as possible. Through years, possibly decades or even longer, of trial and error, making mistakes or just creative thinking a business will have determined the most efficient way to operate. A business knows the most efficient and cost effective ways of doing everything, they have been in the business for a long time and have also had "trade secrets" handed down to them from people in the business before them.

I use film production as an excellent way to illustrate this. Kids today might be so accustom to their digital photographs and digital cameras; but, this is only a new advancement in technology. The rest of us are equally familiar, if not more so, with the old "35mm" film camera. You probably won't use one anymore but that's all there use to be.

If you remember, a roll of film containing twenty-four exposures cost about five dollars. When it comes to producing films, they use exactly the same film. Another thing to add is that in film production, one second of film is twenty-four frames. So, the roll of film you used to buy for your "35mm" film camera is only enough for one second of film. Count that. That's five dollars for every one second of film. Egad man. Clearly when it comes to producing a film, they do not stuff around. They have been making films with "35mm" film for over a century (approx.) and have developed the system of operation over this time to not waste any amount of time; any stuffing around would cause huge cost blowouts.

There's much more to know about the system of operation when it comes to producing films but that in itself is enough to know to illustrate the importance of a business' system of operation. They have been in the business for years and have been learning from all of the people in that business before them. Damn, five dollars for every one second of film. It probably cost even more in the older days too, when film was relatively new technology.

I also wanted to add the words from a song I wrote a few years ago; but, I think I might add something else first. I haven't touched on "Team Work" yet, so why don't I add a little bit about that then? This is something else that might seem like it is directed towards adolescents as well; but, with some of the co-workers I've had to endure in my years I'm not so sure.

Team work is something that is very important for kids to understand when it comes to operating well at their job when they get one. In fact, it's probably something they're going to be asked about at an interview. In fact I did touch on this in my bit about business and how a business can grow from only one person doing everything to having a small team to do everything and then growing to have a team in each area. I don't include any examples of how it is imperative to work as a team to perform and accomplish tasks though. This is probably what a prospective employer is likely to ask in a job interview as well.

My favorite example of how it is not only important to work as a team but also how a task cannot be accomplished without team work is this.

What happens if there is a fire on a ship? How do they put it out? Well, you might be likely to assume that some guys point hoses at it and it goes out eventually; but, this doesn't actually work in the real world. It requires a team. The first man has to contain the flames and heat by having his hose spray which creates a wall of water that flames and heat can't penetrate. The other team members then stream their hoses and water through this first guy's spray. Without the first team member's spraying they are unable to get close enough to the flames to put it out.

Another good way to illustrate the importance of working as a team is my old football analogy. I'm from Australia and "Australian Rules" is the only game of football for me; but, this should remain relevant for most codes of football, even if they're not as good.

When I was working at a well known local restaurant as a kitchen hand and cleaner, I constantly had to leave the sink area to either put away deliveries, fetch something for the chefs, which could take a long time sometimes, or simply clean as part of my regular cleaning schedule to keep the health inspector happy and keep everyone else in a job. That was the role I played. There were chefs to cook the food, waiters to take the food to the customers and cleaners to clean the place and keep the rest of them in a job.

While I was gone I could never trust the waiters to perform the simple task of scraping their plates into the rubbish and then stacking the plates in neat piles. I had to return every five minutes to scrape off plates, place cutlery in the cutlery bin and then stack the plates that had been left strewn about the place into neat piles. I never shut up about it. If I got a dollar for every time I yelled at the waiters to put their rubbish in the rubbish bin or to stack their plates neatly I'd be a wealthy man. It was not just part of their duties and part of the system of operation that dictated that it was the waiters' responsibility to scrape and stack plates into neat piles; it was also a matter of safety.

There was not much room and it was an extremely busy restaurant for its size. I always said that by not stacking plates neatly and relying on me to stop what I had to do to finish their jobs for them was the same as me playing in a defensive role on a football field, kicking the ball to the forward line then having another team member just stand there, not even try to get the ball and make me run up to the forward line to take my own pass, or, taking the mark from my kick then just dropping the ball and walking away.

Imagine that actually happened in an actual game of football, the player that couldn't be bothered doing his part wouldn't have a job for very long.

The moral is that when it comes to getting a job you have to know not only how to do your job and know the system but also know your place and what is expected of you. You have to know what role you are playing in your team and what is the minimum that is expected of you, then exceed it. The more you exceed the minimum the more you are helping out your fellow team members and the more valuable a team member you will be and the more productive your team and business can be.

Now to conclude this unfunny replacement for my disallowed ten or so pages of the word "Barry", I am going to add the words to a song I wrote a few years ago. I can never understand what makes people so arrogant, even when they're absolutely not deserving of being arrogant, or even being proud of themselves. The concept of this song was to ask the questions that need to be asked of everyone. You're arrogant, but why? I think complacence is a scourge, a cancer on the earth, arrogance is even worse and it is rife in this world. I had to ask the questions.

This song is titled "R'd in the A in the P" which stands for, "Raped in the Arse in the Prison". I tried to record this song by myself at home; I only had one cheap microphone to do it with so it sounded terrible and nobody will ever hear it. Yeah, my seven piece drum kit and seven cymbals with one microphone, a cheap one too, terrible. If nobody hears these words because the recording was so awful then these questions are going unasked.

I remember hearing once that, "The only stupid question is a question that isn't asked". I'm not sure who the source of this quote was or from where it originated. Anyway, I wrote these words for a reason and I think it would be a little bit of a loss if these questions were to go unasked, so I'm going to ask them now. Also, I thought the only stupid question was a question never asked; but, that was until I was listening to a commercial radio station one day while I was at work. They regularly paraded out this "Psychic" that people could ring in and ask questions. Why do they encourage these people? Did you ever see "Psychic Sandwich" on Letterman? Hilarious! Anyway, one person rang up and asked "Is my dead mother alright?" Actually it may have been grandmother. This is when my opinion of the phrase, "The only stupid question is a question never asked" began to change. No man, she's dead.

I think it's about time people started to deal with death. Once you're gone, you're gone. All anyone ever **KNEW** was one life and planet earth. It strikes me sometimes that religion was born simply out of the refusal to accept death. If you think about it, "Heaven" reeks of being made up to comfort people in death. "Hell" reeks of being made up to scare people into behaving, because what good was the idea of heaven if anyone old criminal or bad person could get in.

Back to the point, R'd in the A in the P.

The words are:

Who are you?

What are you?

Who are you?

Where are you going?

How are you getting there?

What are you doing?

What were you doing 2 minutes ago?

What were the consequences of your actions from 2 minutes ago?

Are you part of the problem or are you a part of the solution?

Think. Think again. Think again again.

Be smart, think quick. Be prepared. Be alert.

Do good, be polite. Do your best. Be your best.

Exercise. Get strong. Get fast

Be friendly. Be kind. Be generous. Be patient.

Make as many friends as you can.

Know your friends. Know your enemies. Know yourself.

Know your body. Know your mind.

Know the earth. Know yourself.

Understand nature.

Think for yourself. Think again.

Who do you think you are?

What do you think you are?

What makes you that way?

Are you sure?

What to you do in life?

Who do you help?

Are you helpful?

Do you know the solution?

What do you want from life?

What do you want from others?

What do you want from the world?

Who are you?

What do you do?

Know yourself. Know history.

Who are you?

Why are you that way?

Are you really who you believe you are?

Are you really what you believe you are?

Knuckle down. Work hard. Play hard. Rest often.

Communicate. Know communication. Know the media. Know yourself.

Stretch often. Exercise. Get strong. Get fit.

Survival of the fittest.

Are you fit?

Could you catch food in the wild?

How?

Are you smart?

Why?

Are you loved?

By who?

Why?

What were the consequences of your actions from 2 minutes ago?

What are you going to do next?

Why?

Who will that help?

Why?

What are the consequences of your actions right now likely to be?

Ponder. Think. Contemplate. Think through. Think again.

Cause and effect.

Be objective.

Learn something new.

Do some push-ups. Yes now, why not?

Are you successful?

Could you survive in the wild?

Are you fit?

Are you healthy?

Have you made the right decisions in life?

What were the consequences of your actions from two years ago?

Have you made a mistake?

How?

What were the consequences of your mistake?

What were the consequences of your mistakes?

Don't hurt good people. Don't mess with good people.

Be smart. Make friends.

Do something intelligent. Say something intelligent.

Be polite. Be kind. Behave.

Apply your energy to a legitimate career.

Don't just do the wrong thing to rebel, or if it amuses you, because you can.

Why not do the right thing because you can.

You'll make more money.

You won't get bashed

You won't have to constantly look over your shoulder.

You'll stay out of prison.

You won't get raped in prison.

You'll make more friends.

You'll make more money.

You'll make more money.

You can be loved.

Get loved. How? Why?

Who do you think you are?

How did you get that way?

Are you really that way?

What do you do in life?

Who do you help?

Understand nature. Understand history. Be objective. Understand communication. Understand the media.

Do you belong?

To what? Why?

Does this promote intolerance?

Does it promote bigotry, ignorance, racism, segregation or xenophobia?

Does it promote, worse, complacence? Arrogance?

Who does this help?

Why?

Understand humanity. Borders separate economies.

Understand the world. Understand society. Know your job. Know your place. Do your best. Be your best. Push yourself. Give 100% to your work.

Return on your employer's investment.

Are you an investment?

Give 100% to your rest.

Understand your body. Understand your mind. Understand your limits. Understand your place.

Do you actively contribute to the solution?

Have you ever been homeless?

Are you a lucky person? Think again. Think again again.

Take a good hard look at yourself.

Take a good hard look at the world.

Be good. Do good.

If somebody does the wrong thing by you, just go do the right thing by them anyway.

Keep the law on your side.

What were the consequences of your actions from yesterday?

Are you thinking about other people now?

Have you ever?

Why?

Do you want to help the less fortunate?

Why?

How?

Have you considered a job in I.T.?

Would you like to be baker?

Jobs become obsolete.

This is the digital age.

Man created the digital age.

Do you understand global communication?

And, DO YOU WANT TO GET R'D IN THE A IN THE P?

****

BLAKE JOY

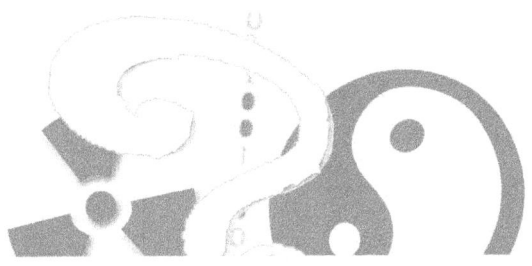

## CHAPTER FIVE
**Your Brain, Brain Exercise, Biomechanics, Pilates, Music, Drink Two Litres of Water Each Day!**

I believe I was going to start with a brand new topic as they are all going to fit together and make sense at the end. Why don't I write about Nutrition and Health for this one?

What have I learnt about Health and Nutrition? (When I ask a question like that I am actually asking myself, it turns out that I write my thought processes as I'm typing.).

Be treat wise, know your DIs. Seriously, do! Your DIs are your recommended daily intake of essential vitamins, minerals, sugar and fat.

There's only very simple mathematics involved in understanding what those numbers mean on all of your food wrappers and packaging, it isn't very hard to understand. If I can do it, you can do it.

The smartest thing you can do is drink water, there will be more on this later; but, I thought I'd write down now just in case I forget to waffle on about it a little between now and the time I finish up the writing of this thing.

- Your daily recommended intake of Energy is 8700 kilojoules.

- Your daily recommended intake of Protein is 47.5 grams.

- Your daily recommended intake of Fat is 73 grams.

- Your daily recommended intake of Saturated Fat is 24.5 grams.

- Your daily recommended intake of Carbohydrates is 284 grams.

- Your daily recommended intake of Sugars is 87.5 grams.

- Your daily recommended intake of Sodium is 2.2 grams.

The trick is to get the balance right. You need to take in enough energy for your daily needs which is, on average, 8700 kilojoules; but, you must also get the correct amount of energy without getting too much or too little of your other essential nutrients. There is not much point to eating only food that is high in fat and sugar; but, low on energy, to get the correct amount of energy you will take on far too much fat and sugar, for instance. If you do this every day you will be taking in far more than your recommended intake of fat and sugar every day to get the correct amount of kilojoules from your food.

There isn't much to it, it's very simple mathematics and should only take a few minutes of looking at the numbers on the back of your food packages to understand. My rule of thumb when it comes to getting a balanced diet is to eat fresh and eat colourful. The colours come from vitamins and minerals in the fruit or vegetables so I always like to have all sorts of colours on my plate.

I highly recommend taking a multi vitamin every day as well. You cannot know exactly what you're eating is made of. You can't know how much of anything is in random food items that you've bought from your local store. I have always thought that you must need to eat a truck load of food each day to get absolutely all the essential nutrients that you need each day. That would throw your sugar, fat and carbohydrate intake out too, so I decided to just start taking a multi vitamin every day. Now I don't have to wonder any more.

Most sweets are sugar and butter. Let's take a lesson in cooking now, or baking.

There is little deviation in the basic ingredients of most desserts or sweets. They all generally contain the same basic ingredients, which are sugar, butter and flour. There's always going to be salt and a raising agent as well. If you want to make a cake, any kind of cake:

Mix butter and sugar until combined, add an egg and some flavouring if so desired (vanilla or almond extract for instance), then add flour, salt and a raising agent, usually baking soda, then add a little milk and anything you want to flavour your cake.

Easy...Cake.

Want cookies? Same thing but no milk at the end.

The point however, is that you can't just fill up on butter and sugar. Fill up on good, wholesome meals with plenty of freshness and colour and then eat up some butter and sugar with a cup of tea later.

Chocolate is also simply butter and sugar. To be exact, chocolate is made of cocoa butter, cocoa and sugar. For illustrative purposes, it is butter and sugar. If you eat only chocolate, for instance, your fat and sugar intake would be extremely high; however, your energy intake will be extremely low.

White flour is an excellent source of energy; you will be taking in much more energy from cakes or cookies than from sweets that do not contain flour.

Even when you get right down to the maths and the figures, good nutrition is still simple to understand.

You need to drink two litres of water each day. If you think you need to keep reading to the end of this book for me to tell you what the smartest thing I think you can do is, you're absolutely wrong. The smartest thing that I think you can do is either drink water, or smile. I read that a person's body loses three litres of water each day. Given most of the food we eat is mostly water, if not all the food we eat, we take in one litre of water each day from our food; if we only take in one litre of water from our food; but, we lose three litres of water every day, what on earth man?

You have to drink an additional two litres of water to replace the three litres of water you lose each day. Do you remember being told that your body is seventy or eighty percent water or something? Well, that would mean that for every day you don't take in three litres of water, your body dehydrates more. If your body is seventy or eighty per cent water or something, then your brain is also seventy or eighty per cent water or something. If you don't replenish the water that you have lost each day, your brain becomes increasing dehydrated by the day as well. So, what yo' think about that Sultana Brain?

I'm not trying to insult anybody; but, for illustrative purposes, think about it. A sultana starts out as a grape, when the grape is dehydrated enough it becomes a sultana. Why would anybody do that to a delicious grape? Sultanas suck, well I don't like them as much as grapes anyway. This is what must be happening to your brain if you're not replenishing all the water that your body loses each day. You need to love your brain, it's the most important thing in your world, it is everything you know, everything you believe, every jaded delusion you have, everything you are, et cetera.

I repeat, you must love your brain, it is everything to you. If you neglect to maintain your brain's health and level of hydration, you simply cannot be operating to your body's natural capacity. Just drink two litres of water every day! Alright? Ya Dig? Get a mean? K?

If all large things are made up of many smaller things and if the large world is made up of many small people, ensuring that these people drink the correct amount of water each day to ensure the correct levels of hydration for their physical and mental capacity would be how one would get on top of these little things of which the large things are made in this instance. One's brain is the most important thing they have, actually, it's probably only as important as any other organs one would have, but it's health, hydration and capacity dictates who you are, what you do, what you're like, how you act, your intelligence, your dexterity to name a few things.

I believe that you also need to exercise your brain to maintain its health and strength like you would with any other muscles or organs. This is where me being a Metal Drummer comes into it. Man, I love The Metal. Meshuggah are my favorite band.

I can't think of anything better than music for stimulating and exercising your brain. Once you begin learning an instrument, you are stimulating your brain every time you practice and every time you hear music. When you practice your instrument you are gaining valuable dexterity as well as hand-eye coordination. I believe that music is, hands down, the greatest exercise you can do for your brain. Computer games are the only thing that come close to music for stimulating one's brain; however, there's nothing in video games to stimulate physical strength or dexterity anywhere other than the fingers. You also don't get to play in bands and perform by playing video games, or gain any of the valuable life skills that also come with being a musician and playing in a band.

I guess I'm going to continue on about music from here, before getting back to the health bit. Team sports are also essential to a child's development.

Do I need a new chapter yet? I'll wait until after the rest of the health bit, which will come after this music bit. I'm enjoying writing something with no organisation or structure. I'm a profoundly organised person, a complete neat freak. I think I've admitted to being a bit of a bureaucrat before so this is a little bit of fun for me. It's important to be neat and I'll explain why I'm this way later. I'm also hardly one to think about or speak about myself, it might not seem like it from this book so far; but, it's very strange for me to see 'I' written so many times.

Music, remember? I am absolutely enchanted by music; my eldest brother was a real music lover when I was growing up and a big fan of the band "The Cure". This really rubbed off on me and I grew up a music lover too. I grew up always wanting to play an instrument and when I was about fourteen I decided to buy a drum set and play in a band with a mate who had been playing guitar for almost a couple of years. I became enchanted with music, it had everything, I loved it. I did it because it was fun; but, it became so much more.

Take a mental journey back through history to a time before music had been invented or discovered or what ever it was. Once upon a time, there was no music. The first instrument is believed to have been the Marimba which pre-dated the Violin by thousands of years. The earliest Marimbas are believed to have been made by women who would place their legs over a hole in the ground; they then placed lengths of wood over their legs and struck them.

If you get right down to the physics as well, you can break up what music is into its components.

Essentially, music is vibration and resonance which is played over time. The vibration is caused by striking a membrane, piece of wood, piece of metal or plucking a string. The resonance is produced by resonating chamber where the sound of the initial vibration is amplified. Drums, for instance, are a cylindrical hollow piece of wood with a membrane pulled tightly over one, or two, of its open ends.

Vibration is caused when one strikes the membrane; the vibration is then amplified by resonating within the hollow cylindrical piece of wood, which is the resonating chamber. An acoustic guitar, for instance, is a hollow body with a protruding neck and strings. Vibration is caused when one plucks or strums the strings; these vibrations are then amplified by the hollow body, which is the resonating chamber. When these vibrations are amplified by resonance and are played over time, the result is music.

Something that can produce a vibration and a resonating chamber are common to all musical instruments, except for modern electric instruments. Electric instruments have no resonating chamber. If you have ever heard an acoustic guitar and also heard an electric guitar with no amplification, the acoustic guitar is much louder because it has its own resonating chamber. Electric guitars use magnets to pick up the vibration, for those not in the know the series of magnets are unimaginatively called "Pick Ups", the vibration is then transformed into an electrical impulse which then travels down a cable to an amplifier which turns the electrical impulse back into a distinct sounding vibration with a speaker. Actually, please excuse me, I meant to write, this electrical impulse travels down a cable, through a fat distortion pedal, then through another cable and into an amplifier. This technology has only existed since the nineteen fifties and is the invention of the late, brilliant, Les Paul.

Musical instruments, like tools, have evolved from the early simple forms of marimbas to the complex electric instruments of today. Imagine a time before music had come into being, then come back to today and take a good hard look at all the love and happiness that has come from music. Music which is simply vibration and resonance played over time.

What does music have to do with health and nutrition? Well, nutrition, nothing; but, health, well, I'm a drummer and the benefits to my physical and mental capacity are greatly enhanced due to my love of music and love of drumming. I'm what is referred to as an "Extreme Drummer", meaning I play really fast metal. It's quite an athletic endeavor. There was a time when I couldn't play at all, of course, I had to start somewhere, knowing nothing, learning and practicing. I started to practice by learning basic rudiments and exercises that helped me to coordinate several limbs at once. My physical strength and dexterity improved and just continued to improve the more I practiced. I can now use all four limbs completely independently of each other. Playing Metal on the drums also keeps you fit. It's a full body workout, pretty much. Your head, neck and face muscles all get to have a go as well; seriously, Metal's really fun.

This takes us to "Biomechanics". What is "Biomechanics"? Well, do you know what "Mechanics" is? A mechanical device is a device that has small moving components that combine to create a larger device, like an engine for instance. An engine has many moving components that all work together to make up the engine. Biomechanics is how all of your muscles work together to create the functions of your entire body. I have studied Biomechanics extensively as a Metal Drummer. There is an optimum way to use your body to achieve that level of fast drumming. Biomechanics is also the way I can learn much from the animals, especially the big cats.

As our bodies have evolved, so too have the animals to be good at different things. Horses are good at running, because they have no defense mechanisms to fight off predators in the wild so they have adapted to run. The big cats are the top predators that have adapted to chase down their prey, so they are also built for running as well. The animals instinctively use their bodies and muscles as nature has intended. Humans don't use their bodies or muscles as nature has intended, only the elite athletes push their bodies to its capacity. Elite athletes like Metal Drummers.

In the wild it is survival of the fittest. You have to be good at fighting or running away to escape predators and survive. The same is true of human society; but, instead of predators it's criminals, unless one was to venture into the natural habitat of large carnivorous animals. Each animal has evolved to be extremely good at evading predators, they simply would not exist today if they had not developed, adapted to their surroundings and become either extremely good at defending themselves against predators or extremely good at running away from predators. I believe that the evolution of all animals is facilitated by the fight or flight response and adaptation to their surroundings and emerging threats.

Your muscles are intended to work together to achieve your body's natural capacity. This is biomechanics. Like the small components of an engine that all work together to create the engine, your muscles all work together to create your whole body. This is how music and drums comes back to health and nutrition.

I stretch my legs, arms and back muscles at least twice each day. Stretching your limbs puts your muscles into alignment with each other, this is called, "Muscle Balance". One can achieve much more strength when many muscles are all working together towards a common cause. Maintaining a good posture is also important, one's muscles are not balanced and one's body is not bio-mechanically correct if one does not have a good posture. To achieve a good posture, raise your hands to shoulder height, push your shoulders back as far as they can go, then push them forward as far as they can go, then take them back about half way. Return your hands to your side. Done, perfect posture. Now your muscles will be working together better.

I have six main stretches that I do, daily at least, to achieve proper muscle balance and biomechanic correctness.

The first is simply keeping my legs straight and trying to touch my toes. I go as far as I can go without straining too much, then I hold it for about twenty to twenty-five seconds, then I carefully return to upright.

The second stretch I do is my groin; I spread my feet to a little further than shoulder width, keep my back straight, keep the bottoms of my feet firmly planted on the ground and bend either knee whilst I keep the other leg and back entirely straight. I bend my knee until I can feel it in the groin muscle on the opposite side to the knee I am bending; I then hold it for twenty to twenty-five seconds.

The third stretch I do is simply taking hold of my foot behind my back side, then straightening out my back until I can feel it in the thigh of the leg that is bent and being held behind me, I hold this for twenty to twenty-five seconds.

The fourth is, placing one hand on a wall, placing one foot behind me and while keeping my back heel on the ground, bend the knee of my front leg until I can feel it in my calf muscles. I then hold it for twenty to twenty-five seconds.

The fifth of these stretches is taking hold of my elbow behind my head, in line with my spine and then moving my hand to be as close to inline with my spine as I can manage. I then hold it for twenty to twenty-five seconds.

The last of these six stretches I do by extending one arm, putting the other arm underneath it and cradling it with the front side of my elbow, I then push down with the arm on top while I push up with the arm on the bottom. Once I start to feel the strain, I hold it for twenty to twenty-five seconds.

If you do this, you should feel fantastic. Your muscles will be totally aligned and balanced. All of your muscles are connected to each other and they all work together. When you stretch your legs and arms, you are also stretching your back and neck muscles. If you have a sore neck, or back, you might just need to stretch your legs, or your arms.

That's how I get back to health and nutrition from drumming. Biomechanics and muscle balance is of the essence when it comes to playing the drums at my level. I need all my muscles working together the way they're supposed to or it doesn't work properly.

Gravity also puts much strain on a drummer's capacity to play. Being able to resist the forces of gravity with correct muscle balance and biomechanics is also extremely important.

Gravity is constantly exerting a downward force on our bodies, if your muscles aren't properly aligned, single muscles or muscle groups will be working on their own to compensate for this downward force. This is likely to create great strain on certain muscles or muscle groups as well as use up a lot more energy. To be straight, a person with a good posture will require and use far less energy compensating for the downward force of gravity than somebody that doesn't have a good posture. By using less energy working against something you can't even see or feel will leave you far more energy for flight or fight, or to simply have more energy to invest in life.

A person with a good posture who stretches regularly will have all of their muscles aligned and balanced, this means that each muscle will work together, from their feet right up to their upper torso, each working only a little bit to compensate for the downward force exerted on them by gravity. It's almost the same principle as "Strength in

Numbers" (Unknown) and "Many hands make light work" (Unknown).

Another thing that is extremely important to one's health is regular exercise. I've read that one should be doing thirty minutes of exercise each day. I exceed this daily exercise requirement by hours. There are many ways to get the exercise you need each day, I don't pay any money for gyms, I've only set foot in a gym once, at a hotel while I was on a holiday in Hong Kong. That was great, the gym was on the top floor of the hotel overlooking the harbour and Causeway Bay, brilliant.

I get much exercise from my work; I have always done jobs that involve hours of manual labour. As long as I'm doing manual labour I'm getting good exercise and I don't have to pay any money for it. This doesn't mean that if you get a job doing manual labour you're going to get an awesome work out. I want the exercise and do this manual labour, involving much running, lifting and repetitive movement as quickly, or efficiently, as I am capable.

I have also incorporated much dancing, which is moving in time to a rhythm, into my work as well to achieve greater fluidity in my movement, which I can speed up and slow down according the demands of the day. The point of all of this is that I don't mind doing hard manual labour jobs, because I want the exercise, I thrive in these jobs because I want repetitive heavy lifting, I want repetitive movement, I want to run around all day because I want the exercise and I love the exercise. If it wasn't for the whole stalking case thing, I wouldn't have to be doing these types of jobs anymore; however, as long as I have to do them, I don't mind because it's great exercise and I get paid while I exercise instead of having to pay a gym and waste my time making up for the exercise that I wasn't able to do at work.

I try to practice my drumming for at least one hour a day. My regular daily practice usually involves plugging some headphones into my iPhone and playing along to Pantera, Fear Factory, the Meshuggah songs I know and other stuff with loads of double kick. For those that are unaware, "Double Kick" is when a drummer plays with two bass drums, or as most people might know them, the big ones on the ground.

Double kick drumming is why muscle balance, correct posture and biomechanics are so important to me. There's an ideal way to play double kick properly, if your muscles aren't balanced and bio-mechanically correct, you're using individual muscles and individual muscle groups too much. These individual muscles and muscle groups become far too fatigued far too quickly and you start hacking it up. The point to this is that I also get much exercise when I practice my drumming as well; I get twice the amount of exercise that is recommended most days by practicing my drums, which couldn't be more fun.

Just for the record, I play a nearly silent electronic drum set at home these days to keep the noise levels appropriate. I didn't always and I seriously annoyed a few neighbours when I was younger. I bought an electronic drum set one day and, well, "Now why didn't I just do this years ago?", I thought. They're a great investment for any drummer, they're essentially a drum kit with headphones and a volume control. If you want to play like me, unfortunately an electronic drum set will only last about twelve months. I've been practicing by hitting rubber pads with drum sticks for quite some time now.

I also do Pilates. I'm quite a fan of the work of Joseph Pilates. The reason for this is that I had the idea to not want to have to pay anyone to exercise. I thought that I could use the downward forces of gravity as resistance to get my exercise. I started researching this, thinking I was the first person to think about it like a bit of a retard, to find out that this is exactly what Pilates is. This meant that I only had to read what Joseph Pilates had already discovered, observed and then communicated. Brilliant! I could spend my time doing something else because Joseph Pilates had already done all the research and study I was about to do.

Pilates is using gravity as resistance; however, there is more to the philosophy of Pilates which I learnt as I studied and practiced further. This philosophy is, well, have you ever heard the song, or heard of the song that goes... "The 'something bone's' connected to the 'other bone'" and so on? This means that if all of your muscles are connected and are supposed to work together, then they all come together in your mid section, your middle abdomen. This middle part of your abdomen is referred to as your "Core".

Your core group of muscles, between your pectorals and your abdominals, your upper abdominals and middle back, are the muscles that work behind all of your other muscles, your leg muscles, your arm muscles, your upper and lower back muscles, your neck muscles, your pectorals and your lower abdominals. Consider any movement you make, with any limb, as a chain reaction of muscle movement that begins from your core set of muscles. The point now is that these core muscles are the foundation on which all the other muscles work, the stronger they are, the stronger the foundation and the greater strength each muscle working with these core muscles behind them will have. On the other hand, the more lame or feeble your core group of muscles are, the weaker or lame the foundation is and each other muscle will not have strong core muscles working behind them.

This is the philosophy of Pilates; it isn't just a way to exercise free. When you move any limb, you're working out and strengthening your core group of muscles, so get moving, stay moving, the more you move and the more you do, the stronger your core group of muscles will become. If you really want to get a strong, solid core, just get on the floor and start doing some Pilates.

I never read much into Pilates. I spent a few hours one night and some of one morning reading up on both Joseph Pilates and his work then never read any further; however, I saw the "infomercial" for "Windsor Pilates" so many times.

When I started to incorporate this into my weekly regime, I began by getting on the floor, I firmly placed my back against the ground and put my hands beside me, palms down. I lifted one leg off the ground and then continued to do anything at all with it. Up and down, side to side, clockwise, anti clockwise, whatever. I then did the same thing with both legs and damn that was some serious stuff. It really works. Damn.

To work on my upper body I tried to remember and replicate some of the things they were doing in the infomercial. I think it was on after Letterman and this was at a time when I would watch Letterman every night, even if it was just for the band. They're awesome. I just love watching absolute professionals doing their work, and doing it so well. FYI…..b. I absolutely swear by a few minutes of Pilates each week now. I get much exercise doing manual labour jobs and playing the drums, so Pilates is just something else I do as well. Having a strong core group of muscles is of much benefit to my physical capacity and increases my capacity to do all of my manual labour jobs and my drumming, quickly, very quickly.

I also like to do some of the basics as well. I try to do at least one repetition of twelve "push ups" every day. I know that there's no repetition if you only do something once so don't write to me about it. Good old "sit ups" are also something I like to work into my weekly exercise regime. My weekly exercise regime that I should be getting back on with, I stopped doing Pilates on purpose to see what the effects were. My core got weak and my physical strength was affected. My abs haven't been quite as hot either. Damn. I have to get back to it now.

If you are doing Pilates or any other exercise for the first time or haven't really done any serious exercise for a while then you might just want to take it easy to start with. That also goes for stretching: start small and ease into it or you might injure yourself. Small steps, the journey of one million miles begins with the first step....you know? Big things are made of many little things. Should you consider heeding any of the stuff that I've had backed up and up and up and up and up and up in my head for decades, consider your goals the big things that are made of many little things. The little things that make up any one goal are the steps you have to take to get there. Take it one step at a time and ease into any exercise or fitness regime you might like to have. You might get hurt. You have been warned.

K. There'll be no blaming of anybody but yourself if you go too hard too quickly and rupture something, or pull something, K? I highly recommend to everybody thinking more about their nutrition and physical fitness, and I encourage everybody to get into a bit of exercise or Pilates; but, take it easy to start with, go at a steady pace.

Make it your next step to better your last performance each time. "The sooner you start something, the sooner you'll finish something" (Unknown). "The hardest thing to do about anything is starting" (Unknown). Are there any more I might be able to add at this point? Lift with your knees and not with your back. Even though I was only joking about that last one, I think that it's heavy things that one should lift with one's knees, if you don't exercise your back it's going to get weak and then it will start hurting.

Don't neglect to exercise and strengthen your back because you were told to lift with your knees and not with your back. If you don't exercise your back, it will become weak and then it might become inflamed and hurt. I think most people's complaints about back pain could probably be explained by the muscles being weak and the pain being due to inflammation. Pilates will strengthen all of your core muscles and make your back strong. On the flip side, it's common to pull up sore after exercising and athletic endeavor, or just by doing physically demanding, hard work. You just can't get out of the pain when it comes to your back. It's going to be a little painful whether you exercise or not. If you do decide to exercise your muscles, it will only create discomfort for one day, then after that it will feel awesome. You'll have a strong back and you'll be able to feel it.

To finish up these several chapters, I'll do my bit about "Pain". Pain is a part of life. It only hurts for a little while. "No pain, No gain" (Unknown). My favorite saying about pain is one I heard while I was inadvertently watching a television program about guys trying to get into the French Foreign Legion, or something, the quote was, "Pain is weakness leaving your body" (Unknown). Do you know how hard you can hit your leg if you accidentally miss your snare drum, or if you hit one of your fingers while you're playing the drums? What can you do when it happens? You can't even make a noise; there are all of these microphones around you. You just have to deal with it and play it off.

Just for the record, getting sweat in one of your eyes when you're playing drums is the worst, there's nothing more painful, you can't stop and you can't make a sound. I absolutely love playing the drums, it has everything. Getting sweat in my eyes was a common thing for me when I played my drums; I had to start wearing sweat bands on my arms and sometime even a head band. It's pretty cool though, nobody's going to give me any grief about my head band when I start playing, it's just a way to keep the sweat out of my eyes. Ouch.

****

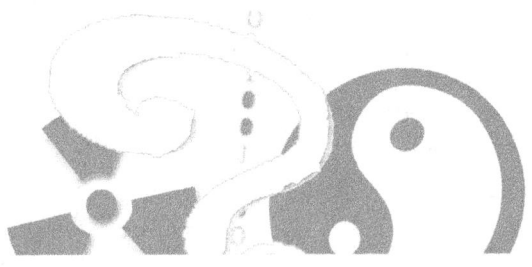

## CHAPTER SIX
### The Media and Objectivity.

This time I'm going to get started on "The Media" and what I've learnt about the media since I began studying it when I was thirteen, when I had no choice. I believe that having a good understanding of the media is very important. Objectivity is so important. Objectivity is so important, objectivity is so important, objectivity is so important, objectivity is so important, objectivity is so important, objectivity is so important and objectivity is so important.

Everything you think you know isn't what you know. Everything you think you know is only what you have read or been told. There's every chance that everything you were told or have read about something could be incorrect and that you have been misinformed. Nothing is knowledge until it is proven beyond any reasonable doubt.

"There's two sides to every story" (Unknown), "Get your facts straight" (Unknown) and "Keep it real" (Unknown) are common sayings, now I'm going to tell you why and how they all came to be.

There's a good film to watch about this matter titled "Body Shots" (1999). The film "Existenz" (1999) is also a good film to watch about this matter. The classic Australian series "Frontline" (1994-1997) is also a great way to get an insight into how things really do operate behind the scenes of a current affairs style television program.

"Media" is what we use to communicate. When we communicate we are imparting, or sharing, an idea or message to a recipient, or audience. To share an idea or message we need to use a medium like speech or gestures. The word "Media" is plural of the word "Medium". This means that anything a person uses to communicate with another person is "Media". This includes telephones, writing, speech, emails, SMS text messages, gestures, signs, radio, television, billboards, semaphore, sign language, smoke signals, newspapers, magazines and posters. "The Media" is often confused with "The Mass Media". This means that when people hear the word "Media" they often think of mediums of the mass media like television, newspapers and radio; however, the media includes anything a person can use to communicate with any other individual.

"The Mass Media" is also referred to as "The Popular Media". Mediums of "The Mass Media" are far more effective at communicating to a large amount of people at once.

"The Mass Media" began with the invention of the printing press. The printing press made it possible to create a template and print many copies of something from its template. These prints could then be distributed widely. Mass production also happened as a result of the invention of the printing press.

As printing evolved and developed, being able to put a communication into a publication that was going to be seen by many people at once made having a press or access to a press worth lots of money. All the newspapers, television and radio networks or businesses make most of their money from selling their medium to businesses so these businesses can get their communication about who they are, what they do and why anybody should care to as many eyes and/or ears as they possibly can.

Buying advertising space during the highest rating television or radio shows is going to cost far more than it would during less popular programs. Television networks work by trying to get as many people to watch their programs as possible to make their advertising space worth more money to businesses. They also try to save money as much as possible, for example, a drama costs a lot of money to produce whereas a reality television program like "Big Brother", for instance, is inexpensive to make, cooking shows are inexpensive to make and travel shows are inexpensive to make, In fact, I'd be surprised if the television networks pay anything at all to produce travel shows, they're ads for hotels and resorts and so forth, it wouldn't be too great of an expense to fly in a small crew to stay at your resort for a few days, even feed them. For the exposure a business will get by appearing on a popular travel show this expense is easily justified.

This is the business end of the mass media and mass communication. Every television or radio network is a business like any other, the same is also true for newspapers and magazines. They are in it to make money and they make money by making people want to read their publication, listen to their radio programs or watch their television programs.

The reason objectivity is so important is that when you're getting your news and information through mass media providers; you're getting your information according to that business and its interests. It's important to remember that there are two sides to every story and you might be getting your information from somebody or an entity that is related to or has interests in one side of an argument. I think people should just listen to both sides of an argument or story and assume they're probably both lying. Remember, nothing is knowledge until it is proven beyond any reasonable doubt. Think logically.

There's every possibility that everything you've been told was wrong, even a lie. The world, even the universe, as you think you know it might exist only in your imagination. Keep it real. You have to be objective. You have to listen. You have to be objective. You have to listen.

Don't ever lie. Lying is the most stupid thing you can do. There's absolutely no point and communication simply can't work properly if you lie. Honestly is not just the best policy, it is the only policy. Lying, just don't do it, it's absolutely stupid, it's the most stupid thing that anybody can do. There's no point lying and if somebody's trying to talk to you about something, just be honest, there's no excuse for lying. I think that's important to add. If you can't stop lying and just be straight and honest, what good are you?

Another thing that is important when it comes to understanding the media, or interpreting the media, is journalists. It is a journalist's job to be objective. The newspaper and television production businesses need to get as many people watching their programs and news as possible, so they need good stories so that people watch their news programs. They invest in journalists to go and report on interesting stories that are likely to make people want to watch, read or listen so that the advertising space during their news is worth as much as possible. Generally they just go about their jobs and report on matters of common interest and big news events in a fair, honest and objective manner; however, there arises a conflict of interest when it comes to journalist trying to make a name for himself or herself and make some money, or more money.

A journalist will often use the popularity of another individual, like a well known sporting personality or popular performing artist in an attempt to report on a story that they believe will be of much interest to the public. It can be like a frenzy sometimes, I think that every time a celebrity is in the news it was because they stuffed up and journalists could not be quicker to swoop on the name to get a story that is of interest, a story that a newspaper, magazine or television production business will invest in so that many people will want to purchase their magazines, read their newspaper or watch their daily news programs. This will make their advertising space worth much to a business trying to communicate with as many people as they possibly can.

Following this rule, journalists will even start stalking these names, who have already appeared in the media for a problem with alcohol or even having a slight mental illness for instance. These journalists know that these people have a problem. They wait and stalk them to catch them in a moment of weakness, so they can then report on it.

How interesting, that sporting personality gets too pissed again, read all about it here. People are pathetic to even use these people for their entertainment.

The people who fall prey to this became well known for being extremely good at something and they worked very hard to get extremely good at something. They might have vices; but, so do all the people that read these things and then look, and talk, down about these people who became well known for being good. The only difference between a well known celebrity having a vice, or bad habit and the people who are speaking down about them is that the people looking down at them, after some journalist had been stalking them to catch them in a moment of weakness, is that these people were never good enough to become known for being good at something, or being good enough at something to make a name for themselves. Too true, right?

You know it....You'd do it. You're a knob.

Just being honest, if that's what you've done, don't lie about it to yourself or anybody else, just accept it, and stop being a knob. Then who are you going to annoy? Who's going to want to hit you then? Keep it shut or keep it positive. Get your facts straight!

Did I mention that this book is being intentionally written with no form or structure at all? Well, any ways, lying is the most stupid thing you can do, pretty much, there's other really stupid things a person can do; but, I think lying is equally stupid as the most stupid of them. Lying always leads to more trouble or further complications. What you think you know about the world could have all come from a lie. This is going to cause problems every time it becomes apparent that what many people think they know is wrong and at the very bottom of it is dishonesty.

Nothing is knowledge until it is proven beyond any reasonable doubt, nothing is knowledge until it is proven beyond any reasonable doubt, nothing is knowledge until it proven beyond any reasonable doubt. Egad man.

I think that these are the most important and significant things to know when you are interpreting the media. Objectivity man!

****

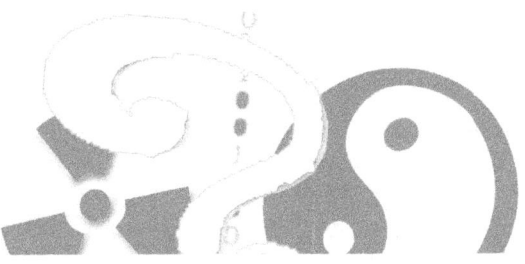

## CHAPTER SEVEN
**The End of the World, The Manhattan Project, The Cold War, WW2, The Nuclear Bit.**

What else is important to life on earth, now? As in December 2012...ohhhhhhhh I'm soooooo scared. I live close to water and I have a little bit of concern in the back of my mind. I'm obviously one to make fun of this Mayan thing while still thinking there might even be reasonable call for alarm. If you live close to the water perhaps? Ah well, apparently Dr. Karl from Triple J said that mathematically it was supposed to happen this morning at nine o'clock. I suppose this is what's going to happen on the twenty-first of the month too. Maybe they mean a new *kind* of world or something because this one could be much better; I think I might have some ideas, one hundred and fifteen pages or so of ideas, so far. There are some stinkers to come too.

I'm beginning to think that I might have to roll a die or something to decide what to write about next. Where do you start? Anywhere, anywhere at all. If there's a job to do, a big job to do, just get to it, start anywhere. The sooner you start the sooner you'll finish.

Now I'm going to do the nuclear bit. I love the entire nuclear thing. I think the whole atomic age and what was learnt is one of humanity's greatest scientific achievements; however, it has its place.

Where did the whole nuclear thing come from? Do you remember that mad adolf rapist of the world guy? Essentially, it all came from what that complete and utter psychopath did. That complete and utter bastard started this massive arms race that has stuffed up absolutely everything.

Before I get on with it I might just make my position regarding hatred clear, because that prick just makes me go there. It is my position that hatred is there and will always be there; but, you absolutely shouldn't go there. You may get pushed there. Just do your best to remain above it, getting pushed there is different. Do your best to not go there, if you get pushed there, it isn't your fault. Play nice. I believe that if somebody does the wrong thing by you, you just do the right thing by them anyway. There's no need to take offence at anyone, just get on with your life, get them out of your mind and out of your system.

This doesn't mean that you don't need to defend yourself against people that are aggressive or hostile towards you, or that I don't think you should defend yourself if you have to. Defence is important. You're allowed to defend yourself and your interests. It's survival of the fittest, you have to defend yourself against any threats that might come your way, or you're toast, buddy.

"Love; but," (Unknown).

"Live and let live" (Unknown).

Any man, or woman, has the power of life or death over any other living thing. It doesn't make you special to have this power, everyone has it. It is then, those that are not able to contain their power over others that are truly the enfeebled, weak and lame.

To get on with it, what we, "The Allies", had to do to stop that insane rapist of everything good led to "The Manhattan Project". "The Manhattan Project" was the course of study and testing that created the atomic bomb, and the atomic age. It's unfortunate; but, we had to make these massive bombs before that insane bastard did. It's even more unfortunate that we had to use them, on people, people that had no say in what their leaders were doing. What an absolute shame, it seems clear that the leaders that want to be belligerent and aggressive are putting their people in harms way, without giving them any say in what is happening in and around their homes. What a needless and tragic loss of life.

The Second World War is something that I have also studied for many years. It's a very important part of history and anybody that wants a clue about the world of today should have a decent understanding of what happened and what the consequences of this war were, so I'll give you the short and skinny of the Second World War, its consequences and then bring it back around to the nuclear bit again.

What led to the Second World War was the First World War and then the Napoleonic Wars before that. That's a whole lot of fighting, keep it in your pants already people, damn. What led to the Napoleonic Wars was obviously centuries, possibly millennia, of people being complete and utter raging, belligerent, warmongering psychopaths.

The First World War was ridiculous. Apparently, according to my research, it started because after the Napoleonic Wars, countries made all of these agreements and partnerships. If one country went into war, another automatically went in as well. One country said, "If those two countries fight together then we fight against them". Then another country said, "If they're fighting, then we're fighting against them". Then several other countries said, "If those three are fighting, then we are too". That, and I think somebody might have been shot or something. World War One, for me, is the perfect lesson on how stupid people can turn the loss of one man's life into the loss of over forty-million lives, or something. Stupid.

As far as I'm concerned, there is no such thing as a world war one hero.

The Second World War happened because after the First World War, Germany was found to be responsible. Germany had many embargoes and sanctions placed on it. The third reich came along and after a while, put that rotten puke bag in charge. That hitler, I refuse to use a capital letter at the beginning of its name, decided it was a divine presence on the earth and started making plans for a new world, of which, that knob's vision of Germania would be its center. It has even been discovered; however, don't take my word for this, that this knob's city of Germania would have sunk because the soil that knob wanted to built it all on was far too soft, apparently. What a Knob! So, after he had finalised his plans for Germania and the new world, the puke stick started either killing people or trying to kill people.

The weapons that Germany was manufacturing were far ahead of their time. German engineering was far ahead of other country's. Their technology was so far advanced of the allies that it really is scary to think of what might have happened, or how the war might have ended if the allies hadn't fought so hard to contain them. I've said it before and I'll say it again, egad man. This is where it comes back around to the nuclear bit. Because nazi technology was so advanced, it had been suspected that they may have had the plans for and may have been developing weapons of great destructive force, weapons the world had never seen before, Nuclear weapons, bombs.

It then became the allies' highest priority to develop these weapons before that absolutely insane whack job did. The allies started a program to develop these weapons that they called "The Manhattan Project". Luckily, we got them before that rotten puke did. It's unfortunate that we had to use them, the blame for this lies with the Japanese command and I contribute the loss of life to their direction and decisions. The Japanese high command of the nineteen thirties and forties knew they were putting their people in harm's way and many were needlessly killed by their arrogance and nonsense.

The findings of the Manhattan Project led to other discoveries, like using the same principle of nuclear fission, or uranium fission, used in the bombs to heat water into super condensed steam and spin turbines to create power. This is how nuclear power is created. Uranium pellets are loaded into a nuclear reactor, the uranium achieves critical mass and a nuclear chain reaction starts. The nuclear chain reaction creates immense amounts of heat. The reactor then has to be cooled down with a constant supply of water so that it doesn't melt, as the water passes through the reactor vessel to cool the reactor it is heated to super condensed steam. This condensed steam has enough force to turn turbines that turn generators that create power.

What's the point of this? I'm asking myself here. No form remember? I'm just waffling on here. To answer myself then, the point is to answer the one thing that I assume many people would like to know, Is nuclear good or bad?

Nuclear is good! The atomic age and its discoveries are one of man's greatest scientific achievements and nuclear power is cheap, clean and safe.

Nuclear is good, nuclear power is cheap to produce, it is safe and it is very clean for the environment, under perfect circumstances. Things go wrong, things wear out, things malfunction, tsunamis mess up all sorts of stuff. Nuclear power is indeed very safe to produce and very clean for the environment, under perfect circumstances.

I'm not simply a 'basher' of nuclear energy because its destructive potential is enormous, I love everything about it, everything but knowing that circumstances might fluctuate in some areas, some areas with nuclear reactors that can explode and release radioactive pollution into the air.

I believe that nuclear energy is the only man made thing that has the capacity to wipe out and make extinct all life on earth. We're slaves to nature and if a mass extinction happens due to natural occurrences, well, there's not much anyone can do about it; but, we can avoid causing mass extinction for ourselves.

It would greatly please me if there was a plan instigated that leads to the phasing out of nuclear reactors over the next 50 years or so in favour of, more expensive, gravity fed turbines or hydro-electricity. There's so much energy in gravity that we can use. There's also so much energy in the currents of the oceans and the tides. I think these are valuable resources for man's energy requirements and probably contain all the energy man could ever need. These are clearly the answers for the world's energy resource demands.

Nuclear energy is a way to create enormous amounts of energy that is also clean and safe to produce, in ideal circumstances. The currents of the oceans and tides contain massive amounts of energy that can be tapped by people for their energy needs and has zero potential for a serious disaster and massive loss of life. There is also infinite energy contained in gravity, when it comes to gravity the word "renewable" becomes redundant. The same is true of tides and currents of the oceans. Gravity also presents zero potential for a serious disaster and loss of life. My ultimate position on nuclear energy and nuclear reactors is that it is the potential for danger that is of greatest concern. While nuclear energy really is safe and clean, it is only safe and clean in perfect circumstances. We have seen what can happen when reactors are exposed to circumstances that are far from ideal. As they say, "An ounce of prevention is worth a pound of cure" (Unknown). No potential for a huge disaster with catastrophic loss of life can exist if the reactors do not exist. I don't believe in accidents, I believe in negligence and stupidity and "accidents" happen all the time.

I love nuclear reactors; I just don't trust people with them.

Haha, people suck.

Be alert!

Come on switch it on!

Take a good hard look at yourself. Who are you? Where are you going? How are you getting there? What do you do? What have you done? What are you going to do? Why do you do the things you do? Are you good at the things you do?

I had one of those ticks again. Anyway, I thought I'd write a little more about the consequences and fall out of the Second World War. I think I covered most of the important bits about the nuclear debate that are worth knowing and worth communicating. I don't think that it is absolutely necessary to get right down to the physics and chemistry of it all.

There's plenty to read about it on the internet if you would like to know more.

Back to something quite heavy again. What happened after the allies put that absolute knob in its propagandist mass murderer place? Well, "The Red Army" was the first to reach Berlin. They came from the East. When the war was over and the third reich was defeated, Berlin was divided up into two, one half was given to America, the other was given to The Soviet Union. Then America and The Soviet Union started fighting. Urgh! The Soviet Union had been spying on America and The Manhattan Project the whole time they were allies in the war against Germany. That's how the Soviet Union got the bomb. America and The Soviet Union compared their sizes for about forty years until the Soviet Union couldn't afford to compare their size with America any more.

The Berlin wall was a wall that communist East Germany had put up to stop people from escaping to democratic West Germany during the Cold War. I will never be able to understand what they thought was good about their regime if they had to build a wall and threaten to use deadly force against people trying to get to West Germany to make them stay. I mean, hospitality man. After the Cold War and the collapse of The Soviet Union, the wall was taken down and Germany became one independent democratic nation.

Some great scientific achievements were made in the time America and The Soviet Union were having a nuclear who is bigger. Everything to do with space travel is all about the Cold War. Unfortunately, more not so great things happened as a result of the Cold War, or even as part of the Cold War, the not so cold parts, the Korean and Vietnam wars.

My knowledge of the Korean and Vietnam Wars is not great, these are things I just haven't studied in great detail, I can't do it all, damn. I'm not even sure what the whole stories were with those wars. I've seen quite a few documentaries about those wars and while I think I understand how the Korean War might have started, all I really know about them is that the two sides are capitalist and communist. I never took sides on the socialist and capitalist debate. If a country chooses socialism why can't we just accept them as a socialist country and befriend them instead of forcing our way on them? I had no say in where I was born, or to what regime I have grown up with and into. Nobody has any say in where they are born. Not many people even have a say in what they believe as a child. You take on the beliefs and regime you were born into.

I don't buy into there being an east and west. I'm only interested in seeing one global community. Nobody in the West had any say in being born in the West. Not many people get to choose what they believe either. You see the world, as a child, as your parents and family saw it. You had no choice in believing what your parents did. They had no choice in believing what their parents did, and so on and so on. This can be continued right back to much earlier times, when very little was known about anything. People did not have knowledge and were left to guessing and speculating. There's every chance that the world as you see it might be built entirely on conjecture and that a person may have been misled when they first began to entertain certain ideas. You might be seeing things that just aren't present on planet earth. You see what you are predisposed to see, you can't trust your own eyes.

Damn, you people have to start drinking plenty of water. Your brain is the be all and end all, it is everything to you, it *is* you, you should treat it as though it *is* you. Drink two litres of water every day, or at least try to drink two litres of water every day. Your brain is a very fragile thing and it is extremely easy to get deluded. That's where the saying, "Keep it real" comes from. It is very easy to become deluded. Again, it is very easy to become deluded, K, deluded, very easy. Nothing is knowledge until it is proven beyond any reasonable doubt. Until an idea is proven beyond any reasonable doubt it is only an idea, a hypothesis, speculation. Here on planet earth we're into keeping it real. Seriously, you have to have your feet on the ground.

To start a new paragraph, an idea is merely an electric impulse in our brain. Perhaps an idea might be several or many electric impulses at once or in a certain series. I haven't studied the brain as far as taking long courses in psychology at university to understand exactly what an idea is. I spent that time studying communications and the media; however, there is much to read about the brain, your brain, available on the internet for perusal or study. The internet is great, I stay away from the social networking media sites these days as the people I was associating with on these networking media sites turned out to be highly undesirable, worse than useless. I only saw them as people who would help me...WRONG!!!

Learn your place, damn. Instead, these people were actually spreading other kinds of words, detrimental to my business. I had to drop them, not one person helped me at all to get a lying spoilt self obsessed little girl broadcasting to the world absolute garbage she had built up in her head out of my life. I had to work so hard to get this girl out of my life, I couldn't speak for myself, so I had to rely on the words of others. I always worked hard, I worked at a pharmacy delivering medicine on my bike as an irresponsible and immature twelve year old. I then began to work at KFC when I was nearly fifteen, I stayed on for four years. I then began an apprenticeship as a Baker, which sucked even though I loved the baking bit of it. Then I worked in a warehouse at Lite n' Easy, a pre packaged weight loss food producer, portioner of, and distributor. I was used to hard work and I was highly experienced and trained. This began to come through and then other people around me started to do the talking for me. I was ninety per cent out of it, then I had a huge result.

People thought my work was exceptional, let's face, no false modesty, it was! I'm awesome! It was only a matter of time. These people saw that I did a good job that made a difference to the business. It turned out to be a massive difference, I think I took one-third of the business with me when I left. I'm awesome, just face it (polishes his fingers on the front of his shirt). Do you think you're awesome? Well, let somebody else tell everybody that, if it's true, people are going to start saying it. Anyway, people loved my work, they knew that they weren't as physically fit or strong as me and that they just couldn't do the job that I did. I've also always been as nice as possible, funnily enough, I wasn't all that nice to these people, I yelled at them all so much, about the same things, every day, but they still loved me. They knew they couldn't do the work I did. Then, one day they found out that I wasn't religious, they couldn't argue.

I live according to the laws of physics, I try to utilise my time to its absolute optimum capacity and I have no time for trouble so I behave myself. I've been in trouble before because I made some stupid decisions and I learnt quickly that I couldn't be bothered with trouble. I like to think that I was smart enough to stay out of trouble; however, trouble found me, because I'm hot, apparently, again, it isn't my place to tell you that.

Anyway, I worked really hard to get that lying lunatic out of my life, except that there remained a few "Random Ferals", as I like to call them, that still listened to it. I had a bit of a breakthrough and made a massive difference to the entire world, man, then people I used to hang around with in high school came back and ruined it all. They got me back in trouble because of the delusions of a lying and very forgetful little girl for three more years. They also did this entirely behind my back and I had absolutely no idea whatsoever that I was even in trouble again, for something I can't believe anybody even took seriously, something I had to have X-ray vision to be doing, and eyes in the back of my head, with X-ray vision.

The internet is still good for information gathering and research. You really have to be careful, these people who came back and got me back in trouble after I not only beat this thing; but, ended up making a massive difference to the world as well, were people I called friends that I loved and cared for. Damn.

I'm still rebuilding after this, tell people to buy my book. Please.

I hate thinking about it...full steam ahead!

Eyes on the prize.

What a waste of time, I'm determined to prove that this is an unfortunate incident that highlights the ignorance and stupidity of the people around me and nothing more. This is just a setback that could have happened to anyone if they were good looking and if such an unexperienced child came along and saw everything they were doing as being about them. I'm determined to get back to having a life that's far better than the one I would have had otherwise, I'm just working away at it right now.

Keep it real. Check yo'self before you wreck yo'self, or somebody else fool.

Keep your brain hydrated and exercise it regularly. I commonly use a game of patience called "Free Cell" to get on, and stay on, the ball. I'm not going to tell you how to play it, except for black on red and red on black. Nobody told me how to play it, I figured it out for myself. Now I average about eighty-five percent wins (it's actually ninety-four per cent at the moment for this edition). It is believed that all games of Free Cell are winnable; however, it is not proven. As I was stating earlier on in the piece, computer games are a good way to exercise your brain and hand eye coordination and music is simply the epitome of awesome brain exercise. Listen to how the bass guitar and the bass drum work together and you'll start to understand, if you listen to any good music that is.

I love Metal. Listening to how the bass drums, bass guitar and guitar work together is very easy to understand when you listen to good Metal. If you don't understand what I'm talking about, listen to some Fear Factory or Meshuggah. Good metal bands use two bass drums to create awesome patterns that the bass guitar and guitar/s follow exactly note for note, they can be very clever about how they do it. Is Metal something you really dislike, even hate? Knock it off, understand that it has its place and it also creates much love in the world that would not be there otherwise. It might not be music that you are comfortable listening to; but, many people just can't get enough of it, like me.

If you don't understand it, cool, just don't say that it isn't good or can't be good because it isn't your style. There's a difference between you not liking something and something not being your style. There's no need for unnecessary prejudice and hatred, say that something isn't your style or that you don't understand it, don't just write it off as being bad and don't just hate on it. Metal creates love, you create hate.

I love a whole lot of musicians and Metal drummers. Metal is just a thing of love for me, don't go hating on it and bringing hatred and prejudice to the table, it's unnecessary and it is your evil.

Also understand the difference between hating something and disliking something, when you dislike something say you dislike it, don't say you hate it, there's a difference. To continue with my bit about hatred and how hatred exists and is always there, you just shouldn't go there, it's perfectly reasonable and acceptable to dislike something. Just understand the difference.

\*\*\*\*

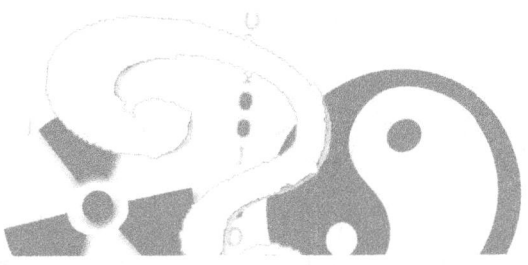

## CHAPTER EIGHT
**Life, Now, on Planet Earth! You Need Skills and Knowledge, Little Business/Large Business, Know Your Flippin' Place!**

I'm going to waffle on about getting jobs and being professional now. I'm running out of things to write, this book must be coming to the end.

So where does the universe end?

Anyway, more about that later. About getting a job then. I think of life as this, you are born and your parents raise you. As you grow up you take more responsibility for yourself and take more responsibility away from your parents, who have been entirely responsible for you since birth. Your development has entirely been the responsibility of your parents so far. Once adolescence comes about you have to start making decisions, you might not be aware of it or even mature enough to know about it, or care, but these decisions are important and they are creating the foundation on which you will build your life. I know this because I stuffed this up; however, it's hard to tell given that I've had an insane girl trying to destroy me for so many years, and had so many ridiculous friends. So, it's difficult for me to say, I also wasn't very good at school. I was about a C average; but, I did get the odd B and A, and D.

My performance wasn't something to be admired or replicated; however, I did choose media studies and ended up pursuing that right up to university and now I have a degree in communications with an advanced diploma in digital television production. That was a big part of what I did during my adolescence and having these qualifications makes a lot of sense. I haven't really been able to get my name and my business out there, in fact I haven't even been able to play my drums professionally with this lunatic. My story is not one that can be used as an average example of what to expect when you finish school and have to move into the real world and get a job.

To get back to the point, I really wish I had taken my selections far more seriously when it came to picking subjects for my course of study in years eleven and twelve. From my experience, I think that what you need to do at about the age of fifteen or earlier is have a good hard think about what you want to do for a living, a good, honest living. Think about the kind of job you would enjoy. Think about the things that interest you, the kind of job that would remain interesting for you, the kind of job that is likely to continue to challenge you.

When you think you have an idea, get another idea and then make everything you do revolve around the first idea; but, keep in mind the second idea. Get on the internet and do some research into the courses that are available in the vocations that take your fancy. Find out the subjects that you will be required to do in your certificate of secondary education to get a place studying your chosen vocation at university.

I was too irresponsible and immature when I was fifteen to fully appreciate and understand this, I just wanted to jump things on my BMX, play my drums and jam. I wasn't really taking life, or anything else, very seriously. I don't think many fifteen year olds do. It isn't really their place to.

I think it's important to communicate this to young adolescents so that they can understand that every decision they make now, especially regarding their path of education and employment, is creating the foundation on which they will have to build their lives later. A teenager should also be around and involved in their chosen vocations as much as possible, They should get a little bit obsessed with it.

If you choose something like television production, you should concentrate on a specific area like being a director or being a camera operator and just stick with that until you get a job doing whatever it is you decided to concentrate on. If it may seem like this is irrelevant to you if you are well and truly past your teenage years, it isn't, tell your nearest teenager. Also tell them that they might think they're grown up and that they have awesome lives; but, they don't, get over it, most people did the same thing when they were a teenager. Tell them that their parents probably had the same life when they were teenagers. They can start thinking like that when they're twenty-five, their brains are fully developed and they're actually people and not teenagers.

I'm going to get down to business to explain this next bit. A business begins when a person or group of people decide to begin trading their skills and/or tools to people for money. Every business starts small and has started small. Each business has in common communication, skills, knowledge, tools, supplies, suppliers, customers, staff, a point of contact between the business and customers or potential customers, potential customers, advertising and hospitality.

The communication involved in business includes; communications with customers either in the flesh or by telephone or email. Communicating to potential customers, which is another way of saying advertising, marketing or promotion. I'm never sure which one of those three words I should use when it comes to writing it down so I'll just use all three this time, they're all the same thing, it would be like writing the new media digital media convergence media.

I haven't written anything about the new media yet, damn, there must still be a bit to come then.

The other communications involved in business is communicating with suppliers, communicating with bureaucrats, as well as any internal business communications including signage around the work areas, memos, rosters, inductions, contracts, training material, on the job training, checklists for projects or maintenance and the business plan.

*The skill and knowledge* means, the skills and knowledge to be able to render a certain service.

The supplies need to be outsourced. Outsourcing supplies requires communicating with a supplier. The supplies also need to be stored, safely and usually in a small area.

The rest of the things I've listed about what all businesses have in common is communication work. A business wouldn't have customers without communication because nobody would know it was there or what services it offers. Nothing happens in business without communication, communication ties all aspects of a business together to form one finely tuned machine.

Business communications is actually my chosen field these days, I had to choose a more specialised area of communications to concentrate on, I knew I could save any business money or increase their productivity and/or customers with nothing more than communication *so* I decided to take on business communications as my chosen specialty. This is where I want to invest most of my time and money. I know I can save any business money and/or help them attract and handle more customers, it's just a matter of getting it together, getting out there and convincing them.

Any money a business spends on having its communications analysed is going to be a worthwhile investment. A business should see all the money they have invested in having their communications analysed by a man obsessed with business communications come back to them again, unless a business' communications are already flawless. I even reckon that having a business' communications analysed and being told by somebody that has studied business communications for many years that the business' communications are flawless would definitely be worth knowing, definitely worth paying for to know, worth paying me to know, you know?

Moving on, when a person starts a business they will most likely take on all the work required to render a service and all the communications work involved in running the business too. For illustrative purposes I will explain this next bit assuming that one person has started a business on their own. This person I will refer to as "The Boss".

To start a business, the boss will need the skills and knowledge required to render a service. The boss will also need money to buy, or lease, and amend either a premises or a vehicle to establish a physical point of contact and a production space if one is required. Assuming the boss has already achieved the skills and knowledge through his or her education, either tertiary education or an apprenticeship, or similar, the boss will then have to establish communications with a bank to get money, unless they're seriously loaded. This will require a business plan, a good business plan.

Just for the record, you can get great business plan templates from the internet if you're starting a business, or planning to start a business. The Northern Territory government website has a really good one to help people start businesses. I assume they provide the service for Northern Territory residents, I can only wonder if they're so tight they would take exception to people residing elsewhere using their business plan template. I certainly hope they're not because that business plan template has been an extremely valuable resource for me.

A business plan is so important for a business. A business plan is communications work that forms the spine of a business. The business plan develops and grows like the business does, I love it. A business plan forces you to think about everything that is important to address when you start a business. Nobody will lend you money unless they know that you have a solid business plan, have thought about everything and can ultimately pay them back.

Let's assume that the boss was successful in getting the money that he or she needed to lease or buy and amend a vehicle or premises. The boss will also need money to promote the business, or else nobody will know it exists. The boss will, so far, have achieved the skills and knowledge to render a service, established communications with a bank to get the money he or she needed, purchased or leased and fitted out a premises or vehicle and then communicated to potential customers about the business' existence, the services it renders, contact details, address if necessary, possibly a promotion and possibly something about rates of payment for services rendered, or to put it bluntly, why anybody should care about the business and the services it renders.

Traditionally, using introductory specials will persuade potential customers to patronise a particular business over its competitors. The aim is to get people to try out your services cheaply, do an awesome job, be super friendly, be super cost efficient and actively care about getting customers the best value for money and have them want to patronise your business again, even if they have to pay as much or nearly as much as they would to a competitor. They might even begin recommending your business and/or talking about their experience with your business. I've discovered that you're not going anywhere unless you're prepared to do a bit of work, quite a lot of work, either free or for far less than you want. You have to work up to getting paid what you want, reasonably, for the services you render.

Anyway, to recap slightly, the boss has now learnt the skills and knowledge, has a premises or vehicle, has established communications with suppliers and has attracted customers with advertising. Now the boss has to be present at the point of contact between the business and potential customers so that he or she can establish communications with potential customers that are trying to establish communications with the business. K. The boss can then take a booking, render the service and take payment for the service. The potential customer has become a customer, a valuable customer, your bread and butter. Fool.

Should the method of an introductory special or alluring promotion prove to be successful for the boss, he or she will probably have more customers wanting to patronise the business and have more demand on his or her hours than hours he or she has to provide, Especially with all the communication work involved.

The boss will require another person to take care of the essential communications work outside of rendering a service, so that the boss has more hours available to render the service. The boss is investing the business' money into the skills and knowledge of an individual to be able to take care of the tasks that need to be done and be able to perform these tasks autonomously because the boss will be out and too busy rendering the service.

Just to make things clear, an investment is when one spends money on something expecting to make a return, put simply, part with some money for a while and have more money come back. This brings us to "Significant Risk", did I even write that all businesses have risk in common too? Never mind, I'll write it here then, I can't think of everything, you know that this book deliberately has no structure or form and that I'm just getting it out, otherwise I think I'll drive myself insane or waste years trying to organise and structure all of this. Writing it all out and hoping it will all add up and make sense at the end is the only plan.

Significant risk is knowing that when you invest your money into something, hoping you will get more back, you might get less back, or none back. When a business takes on an employee, the boss is investing his or her money into them. To put yourself ahead in the world, make sure that when a business invests in you, you're an awesome investment. Make sure that a business will make more money when it invests in you than it would if it invested in anybody else. You can do this by learning your place. A place for everything and everything in its place, that includes you. Learn your place.

If you work for a business then you are an investment for that business, your knowledge, skills, tools, physical strength, attitude, intelligence, mental fitness, efficiency, to name a few things, are all being invested in by a business and your place is as an investment for a business. This entire bit about business is all about helping people not just understanding their place; but, knowing that it is important to be in their place, because when things are not in their places accidents happen.

When one knows one's place, they know what is going on around them.

Back to business, it's hardly likely that a business will have such a great response from some introductory offers and good word of mouth that it will keep them in business with enough work to keep making money and afford to employ another person. The boss will continue to have to invest in promoting the business and make more people, or in business, "Potential Customers" want to patronise the business. This will require reminding people that the boss' business exists and offering further special deals to entice them to patronise the boss' business over his or her competitors.

A business will, or should, always be looking to grow, otherwise it will be destined for obscurity. A boss will grow his or her business by promoting it with special deals to entice customers. The business can then develop a rapport with these new customers and hopefully build on their good word of mouth by doing an awesome job and caring about providing customers with the best value for money that they can. The business might develop a good reputation.

To continue to grow, the boss will only have so many hours that he or she can render a service, if the business wants to grow the boss will have to invest more money in somebody that also has the skills and knowledge to render the service. A person that has the tools as well would be highly desirable to the boss at this point, probably more so than somebody that doesn't have their own tools. The boss is then investing in this person, and his or her tools, to be able to render the service to the high standards that it has had this far to achieve its good reputation.

The more money that the boss invests in advertising and promoting the business, the more people are likely to be interested in patronising the business, should any deals, promotions or past pleasant experiences with the business entice them. This will mean that the boss will probably have to invest in another person to communicate with customers and potential customers. This means that the boss will then invest in somebody to be polite and friendly when they're communicating with customers or potential customers, to maintain, continue or enhance a good, friendly and professional reputation. The boss might also have to invest in yet another person with the skills and knowledge to render the service too and yet more people to communicate with customers and potential customers.

For illustrative purposes, the boss will now have a team. The team will consist of the boss, whose job it is to render the service, a team member to answer telephones and respond to any other incoming communications, a team member to do the rest of the communications work involved and two other team members, two skilled professionals, preferably with their own tools, that have the knowledge and skills to render the service to the high standards that will continue, enhance or achieve a great reputation for the business.

A business can continue to grow from here, if the boss wants more customers he or she can invest more money in advertising and promoting his or her business. The boss will then require more hands, mouths and minds to answer ever higher volumes of phone calls and incoming communications and to render a service to increasingly more people. The boss will also have to invest in more hands and minds to perform an increasing amount of communications work.

The same basic components of a business remain the same regardless of how big a business is. A business' size is determined by how many employees it has, that is, how many people it has invested in to perform the basic components that all businesses have in common. If the boss wants yet more customers he or she can invest more money in advertising. By now there might be a considerable amount of advertising and promoting to do, so the boss might invest in somebody who studies marketing, advertising and promotion to take care of this work. The boss might invest in several. This will mean communicating to more potential customers and having an even higher volume of phone calls and other incoming communications. The boss will have to invest in people to take and respond to these incoming communications as well, and so on.

The business can continue to grow until it is a big business and has not just a small team, but a team for each component of the business. A team to advertise and promote the business, its brand and its deals, a team to answer all the telephone calls, a team to render the service, a team to take care of all the internal and external communications other than promotion.

A business can go from being one person doing everything, to a person having a team to perform each component of his or her business. So, what do you do? What's your job? What's your place? Your place is being invested in by a business to perform a task, even if it's just answering a telephone, with the high standards that will give the business and brand a good reputation.

Either way, you're a team member, you're a component of the fluid functioning of a business. What's the least you have to do to make sure you're doing all that is expected of or required of you? What's the least you have to do so that another team member doesn't have to finish off your job for you and probably want to kick your arse? Do you ever think about your place? Where is your place? What is your place? Have you ever thought of yourself as something a business was investing in and expecting a return on?

I think I have the critical points about business down, if not I guess you're going to have to hire me to answer questions at your next staff training and discipline endeavor. Get in touch at Blake Joy.com!

\*\*\*\*

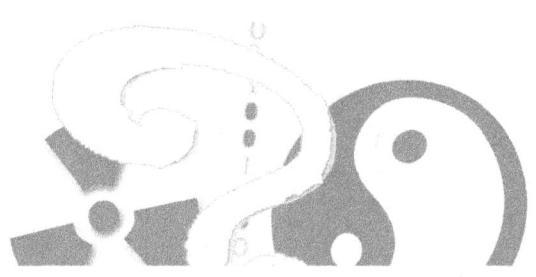

## CHAPTER NINE
**The History of Society, Tools and Engines.**

I'm going to start this with the history of civilisation and the history of society. Get yourselves a nice comfortable spot and relax. This is the history of society as I see it; as it adds up, as it makes sense.

All anybody *knew* was earth, one life and the laws of physics. Human beings are incredibly intelligent beings. The human brain is, beside nature itself, the most awesome and powerful thing that has ever existed. In your head is one of the most advanced and amazing things that has ever existed. Do you think about your brain? Do you think about the health or strength of you brain?

You have to love your brain! It's awesome.

It is believed that human beings were predators; however, it is also believed that humans may have been scavengers. Once upon a time early forms of human beings had to hunt and gather their food. Human beings had the intelligence and dexterity to start using tools to defend themselves against other predators and to help them hunt and gather their food. Human beings also had the intelligence to take another critical step towards society as we see it today. This critical step is farming.

There must have been a point in the development and evolution of man and society when one man made the observation that the food they were hunting and gathering were biological beings that reproduced the same way humans did. It would then be possible to, instead of hunting an animal and eating it, catching several animals and containing them. Instead of having to hunt and gather daily for each meal, people could simply contain animals and have them make more food in their containments. Farming is the foundation of society as we know it. Once farming had time to develop, which would have taken quite a few generations, I suppose, human beings wouldn't have had to hunt and gather anymore.

Humans would have also had a long time to learn which plants they were able to eat and not get sick from. They would have contained and began to farm these as well. They may have been farming plants before they began farming animals, who knows?

Because of farming, human beings that have been doing little else than hunting for food didn't have to do all they had to do anymore.

I'm not sure where the development of tools began; but, it makes sense to me that these human beings had to defend and shelter themselves. Not having to hunt for food anymore would have given early humans the time to develop and invent tools from natural resources to defend themselves from predators as well as make shelter. If you take a good look at everything around you today, it is made from either a plant, an animal, or from metal. These are all things that were available to human beings at any time.

Since this time, it appears that man's tools have continued to develop and evolve, there have also been many crucial developments that have paved the way from the early days of farming to society as we know it today, the invention of the wheel, for instance. I'm going to talk about the invention of the engine, or is that, the development of the engine?

Once upon a time there was no such thing as an engine. An engine is a mechanical device that rotates a shaft. Our entire society is built on engines, the industrial revolution was the product of the invention of the steam engine by James Watt. It's amazing to think about the potential of simply having a shaft rotating, and using it. The entire development of engines is simply making better ways to rotate a shaft. Do you know what a water mill, or wind mill is? You must know what their components are. Water mills have wheels with paddles that are rotated by the flow of water they are submerged in. Wind mills have a kind of wheel with sails that use energy in the wind to rotate a shaft. Horses and other capable animals were also domesticated and used to rotate a shaft. Man learnt that this rotating shaft could be used for many, many things. This is the principle of an engine, which is simply a tool that rotates a shaft.

The invention of the steam engine was a massive deal. I've heard that the steam engine meant that for the first time a shaft could be revolved so quickly that it had to be geared down for practical use. The industrial revolution is what followed and was what happened when man achieved being able to spin a shaft that quickly. Brilliant.

Steam engines were also put onto large boats and had large propellers attached to them, they had wheels attached to them for land bearing vehicles too. Imagine what this must have done when it came to the expansion of communities. Think about the distances people were able to travel with ease, quickly with a steam engine. These distances had been travelled before and trade, which is communicating and sharing things, had already been established much earlier; but, it took a long time to get anywhere relying on sails or oarsmen. I reckon the steam engine was as important as the invention of the wheel.

"Why didn't it end with the steam engine if it was so good?", you will probably not be wondering; however, I will assume you are anyway. As a matter of fact, I can't continue the story if I don't assume you're wondering that. Because, advancements could still be made. From the steam engine it became about spinning a shaft increasingly quickly using smaller components and not having to dig up and burn so much coal all the time. The next step in the development of the engine was the internal combustion engine, like you have in your car. We have come a long way since we used horses to pull carts. We have come a long way since the invention of farming.

Honestly, if you look around all you're going to see is man, his tools and nature itself. An engine is a tool, a car is a tool, a house is a tool, a spanner is a tool, a computer is a tool, a bookcase is a tool, a filing cabinet is a tool, tables and chairs are tools, if you think about what a tool is then society is man and his tools. Society exists in nature. Just for the record, I hilariously misspelt "car is a tool" in the first draft, the "T" is right next to the "R". A cat isn't a tool. A cat is of nature. A symbiotic relationship can exists between humans and cats, some cats, small ones. Cats remain a part of nature, like dogs, even domesticated ones, if we feed them they love us, in a way, sort of, or something.

Man started with nothing except four limbs and an awesome brain. Humans began using things available to them in nature, like sticks and rocks, to hunt and gather food, defend themselves from predators and shelter themselves from the elements. These tools have developed over centuries and millennia and have become more advanced and more complex and they have reached the point of development we see today, today being the digital age. The entire digital age is simply made up from things we dug up out of the ground, what a great time to be alive.

Actually, the atomic age was also what people discovered about things that were dig up out of the ground. Come to think about it, I suppose space shuttle and rockets would be made entirely out of stuff that was dug up out of the ground. The steam engine was also made of stuff that was dug up out of the ground, it was also powered by coal which is dug up out of the ground. Wow.

I'm not quite sure how this next bit fits in exactly but when I was redrafting this book yet again it was just here and I'm still not quite sure how I got here.

Anyway, today it's January 2013. That was fun, let's do it again. I thought it would be hilarious if I wore a bicycle crash helmet on the twenty-first of last month. The day a Mayan prophecy had, many many years ago, declared to be the day of the end of something. I was never quite clear on what it was the end of, or supposed to be the end of. What was with the sequence of numerals 21-12-2012? Wouldn't 21-12-2112 be more like it?

"21-12-2112" is the Australian way of putting it, I believe that in other countries the month occurs before the day, making it "12-21-2112". Perhaps?

Well, we had all start getting along and working together as one global team towards a common cause. This common cause is, of course, not being annihilated by nature or ourselves, or aliens, or Chuck Norris if he turns bad.

****

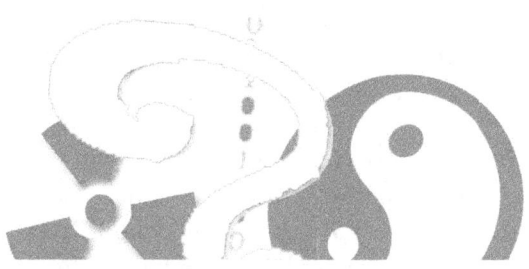

## CHAPTER TEN
**The New Media and Drive Your Car Like You're a Sane Person That Cares About Anything Other Than Yourself and What You Want!**

What happens when you cross a chicken with a hare? Not sure, chicken hare? What happens when you cross an elephant with an insurance salesman? Not sure either. What happens when cross a computer with "The Media", not to be confused with "The Mass Media"? The answer is, "Convergence Media". Convergence media is also known as "Digital media" or "The New Media". Do you remember what "The Media" is? Do you remember the difference between "The Media" and "The Mass Media"?

Communicating with somebody using a digital device is using "The New Media". "The Mass Media" began with the invention of the printing press by Johannes Gutenberg. "The Media" had existed for centuries before the development of the computer. All media that existed before the digital age and are not digital media are now referred to as "The Traditional Media". Nowadays, the internet is heavily used and popular websites have become great places for businesses to have their message and name seen by many people.

I'm surprised there is quite little to add about the new media. I love the new media, I did media studies every year I was at high school, all seven of them, I was heavily into media studies from a young age. My brothers and I also had an Atari and a Commodore 64 as kids. It was great, I was watching the digital age develop right in front of my eyes. I watched the internet come from something brand new when having a modem was like how having a colour television must have been in the day. There was nothing there, practically nothing anyway.

I had been watching the development of computers and the digital age since the first Atari my parents bought for me and my brothers one Christmas. I had been watching the internet grow since the time people had not even heard of a modem, the inter-what now? I was watching the internet and digital age develop all while I was studying the media. Then, I saw something amazing, the digital age, the internet and the media all converged into a whole new world of media and communications. They called it "The New Media", "The Digital Media" and "Convergence Media". That was a pretty cool experience.

What's important about the new media is that the new media is how any person anywhere on earth can now instantly establish communications with anybody else anywhere else on earth, pretty much. Not only did I watch two childhood fascinations come together to create something entirely new and different, I also saw the world become one community, united by instant global communication.

Somehow it came down to me to lead this global community. I just had to open my mouth didn't I? I just had to open my mouth and study communications and the media since I was a kid and know a whole lot about communications and global communications. Didn't I?

Well, anyway, there should only be two denominations in this global community, those jamming to the funk and those dancing to it. What makes any two people different? Colour doesn't make a difference, it's what they have been told and what's in their heads.

Nothing is knowledge until it is proven beyond any reasonable doubt.

This book must be coming to an end, I can only think of three more things to write about before I finish up. These are big parts of everybody's lives today. Actually, I haven't written anything about aeroplanes or jet travel either.

BLAKE JOY

Aeroplanes are also one of man's tools. They have extended the reach of man and man's capacity to travel greater distances quickly and greatly extend communities. The invention of jet propulsion made global travel easy, reasonably inexpensive and accessible to many. This jet propulsion technology and relatively easy global travel made it possible to do all the ground work required to achieve instant global communication using the internet and convergence media.

Another one of the things I have yet to write about, that is also a big part of everybody's lives, is driving. Drive smart, drive sensible, drive like a sane person, drive like you care about your life and the lives of people around you, drive like you don't want to get a fine, drive like you don't want to have to pay more than you need to for your insurance. There are a few things I really have to bring to people's attention. Common mistakes I see drivers making all the time.

Keep left unless overtaking. There are a few reasons for this. If you want to keep it slow, or chilled, then drive in the left hand lane so that people that want to drive a little quicker can easily get past you on a four lane road, that is two lanes one way and two lanes the other way.

Furthermore, people need to make right hand turns and should easily be able to do so without worrying about being rear ended by another car that should not have been in the right hand lane anyway,

160

especially if somebody needs to make a right hand turn after a bend. People also need to make right hand turns from side streets; this is made much easier if the cars are all in the left hand lane where they should be.

You also just have to relax when you're driving, the road is a dangerous place to be, sixty kilometers an hour is also a dangerous place to be. It doesn't seem like it in the comfort of your car with your comfortable seats, suspension and modern conveniences. Just relax. I find driving a whole lot of fun when I keep it safely within the speed limit and try to drive perfectly. I like to keep my car perfectly centered in the lane at all times, even when transferring into slip lanes, paying perfect attention to what is going on around me, always staying left and never crossing a solid white line. Roads simply aren't a place to play.

This next bit is something that I'm certain is going to be difficult to communicate to adolescents. I can see how a kid who has only recently obtained its license and has its own car would want to feel the power of its car and experience driving at dangerous speeds because they can now. Their engine is the most powerful thing they have ever had, it is the most power they have ever known, it is likely to be the most power they will ever know, and they are tempted to use this power. My advice to kids is to get good at a musical instrument or a sport, besides I'm telling girls that there's nothing cool or powerful about a guy that can depress his car's accelerator a few inches rapidly.

I see these kids with their hotted up cars and their big V6 engines, making way too much noise for quiet suburban streets, and I think, "That engine is the only power they will ever know, and it was made by other people". They've bought the little bit of power that they have after it was manufactured in a factory by labourers. Damn you kids suck. It's a little bit embarrassing. The levels of noise would be acceptable in an industrial environment.

I reckon, let these kids rev their engines loudly if they really want to, somewhere the noise level is acceptable. If kids want to drag race their cars they can, I'm sure there are plenty of ways a kid can get its hotted up car onto a track and race against his mates who also have hotted up cars. They each want to open it up, figuratively, and see what it can do. If a kid wants to feel the power it has under the bonnet of its car, it should be allowed; however, they should do this at the appropriate time and in the appropriate place. I'm sure there are plenty of events that anybody can enter and see just how much power their car has and even race against their mates. If there aren't any, which would surprise me, why don't these kids get onto making some arrangements to make it happen? Then who are they going to annoy? Who's going to want to kick their arses then? Then, they will actually be making a legitimate sport of it, and I'll tell girls to dig that.

There are a few other things about driving, proper road use and decent driving etiquette. Indicating is communicating. You can take this right down to semiotics. A flashing orange light is just a flashing orange light; however, when a flashing orange light is on the side of a car, motor bike, truck, or similar it becomes a signifier. What is being signified is that the operator of a vehicle with flashing orange lights on its side is about to maneuver the vehicle in the direction of the side the flashing lights are on. To put it another way, a driver is about to turn. If indicating is a way to communicate to other road users that you are about to turn, what's the bleeding point of indicating only meters from the juncture that you intend to turn? HUH?? Also, what's the point of not indicating at all?

Another thing is that one should always indicate before they begin to break. This was one of the first things my driving instructor told me when I began taking driving lessons. Indicate that you are going to turn BEFORE you begin breaking to slow down for the turn. It's important to think about the people around you, they don't know what you're thinking and you have to communicate to them about what you are thinking otherwise they will never know.

Four wheel drives are too big and far too dangerous, you shouldn't park your big four wheel drives, or similar sized vehicles, close to an intersection, unless it's made of clear Perspex, which it isn't. If a car is too big and parked too close to a corner, any car turning out of that intersection will gradually have to ease further out into traffic to see if there is anything coming and see if it is safe to pull out of the intersection. This means that a car has to pull out into traffic to see if the traffic it is pulling out into is there or not. Dude. You can't just think about yourself exclusively. You have to think about other people, especially on the roads. You have to take some things seriously sometimes, especially on the roads.

Also, don't park with your headlights on in the dark, it is confusing for motorists either coming towards you or pulling out from a side street. It's difficult to tell if a vehicle is moving or not if it is parked with its headlights on. Indicate if you're parked on the side of a road and you intend to pull out from a curb.

****

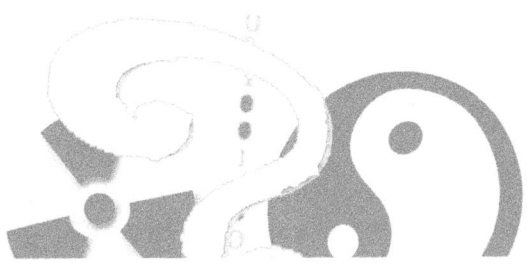

## CHAPTER ELEVEN
### More Music, Consumerism, Commercialism.

Now, what is another thing that is also a very big part of people's lives that I haven't written about yet? Wait a second, I did write about it. Well, anyway, it's music. I just didn't write about this side of it. I haven't written anything about commercialism or consumerism either. I haven't once written, "The lowest common denominator" either. I guess there might still be a little left in this book after all.

I'm enchanted by music, I love it. Once there was no music at all and now we have all of this, all of this love. I'm speaking of good music. I'm not just a massive Metalhead that listens to Metal and nothing else. I love music. I love Metal. I love any good music. I love all sorts of different music. I don't play metal on my drums exclusively. It doesn't matter how quickly I can play my drums, my Breakbeats and Latin could always do with some work. I constantly have to go back to basics to

165

make sure I'm getting on top of all the small things that come together so that I can play the drums quickly.

You never stop learning and you can always be better, perfection doesn't exist. I listen to, love and play all sorts of music. I studied Jazz comprehensively for many years, during this time I didn't want to hear any music I had already heard before. I got over it when the Metal started coming back to me in a big way. I'm a Jazz drummer too, depending on who's asking. I love playing Jazz and Blues on my drums and I think I got quite good at it because playing Jazz or Blues on drums is much quieter and I could play much more without annoying anybody too much. You can't do this if you're a Metal drummer. To be professional about it, a drummer shouldn't play their drum set very often at home if they live in a quiet suburb, especially in a small modern estate with small blocks of land. Ideally, you should practice with an electronic drum kit, which are a great investment for any drummer, when you're at home and then hire a room at a rehearsal studio when you want to unload on a proper drum set. Who are you going to annoy or infuriate then?

I also like listening to and playing Jazz, Blues, Jazz fusion, The Funk, Breakbeats, Trance, Latin, really chilled out ambient music and more. I even dig a bit of Classical music sometimes. Just as I wrote about Metal, don't knock it until you've tried it and understand it. Classical music is great, sometimes. The trick is to just relax and close your eyes, then relax again, and then again, then listen. I love hearing the arrangements of all those traditional string and wind instruments. I love hearing them all working together to create massive pieces of music that are so rich and complex. Just sit back, close your eyes, relax and listen to the instruments, let them take you on a mental journey. If you don't like it, do something (intelligent) that you do like, just don't knock anybody that does enjoy it for what it is. I also enjoy listening to and playing a bit of "Punk Rock" and "Softer Rock" styles of music too.

Another thing I like is a person pushing their limits, like elite athletes. I love music that is different, that is produced by a musician that wants to try things, discover things and do things that haven't been done before. Someone pushing the limits and trying different things, like nomads. I also love people pushing the boundaries of their physical capacity, this is what the allure of Metal really is for me. Metal is listening to people using every muscle in their body, every ounce of their strength, and every bit of their intelligence to produce amazing music. I just feed off their energy. I feel Metal in every muscle and it makes me want to play my drums with everything I have. Actually, it makes me want to do everything I do with everything I have.

Now go and listen to what's allegedly hot on your average commercial radio station. You should find that it is hardly ground breaking, hardly pushing the limits of human endurance. It's pretty weak quite frankly. You generally get the odd good or catchy song; but, usually it's hardly music at all. There might be a little bit of music to it, but it isn't music. If this doesn't make much sense to you it will after I explain this.

Have you heard the saying, "Sex Sells" (Unknown Source)? Well, sex sells better than music does. Funnily enough, I don't think it's because good music doesn't or wouldn't sell, it's that record producers would rather not take the risk in trying to sell good music. Do you remember the part about a business' significant risk? Well, sex is sure to sell, this is how a record company minimises its risk. They're using sex to sell, basically, crap music to you. I think it has even got to the point were a record company will just hire a model and make him or her sing a little bit and use their attractiveness and sex appeal in music videos and posters to sell their records.

That's basically music for me in a nut shell. I want to be inspired and I want to be energised. I refer to Metal as being "Vitamin O". "O" for "Obzen", a song by Meshuggah which is honestly my favorite song right now. I love it.

I think it's time to start finishing up this book.

Now, for the last bit, "The Order". Giddy-up!

\*\*\*\*

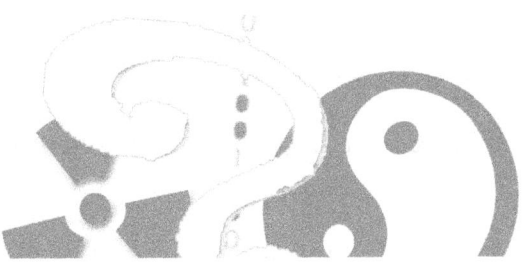

## CHAPTER TWELVE
### The Order!

If we are ever going to achieve an understanding, loving and peaceful global community we are going to require order, rules and regulations that apply to everybody on earth. There should be no more denominations, only inhabitants of earth that are all bound by the same rules and laws of common decency.

Every person must know their place and remain in their place. The global community needs a system of organisation. The global community also needs a way for people to know their place, understand their place and be in their place. I think that there are three rules that are crucial for all people on earth to follow. These are:

• You can't physically hurt anybody unprovoked and without it being in self defence.

- You can't interrupt or impede on anybody's productivity and earning capacity.

- You can't mess with anybody's money, which includes wasting or stealing.

I think these three rules create a solid foundation to begin with.

On top of these simple guides I think it would be beneficial for society in so many ways to provide a system, an order, where people are constantly moving to actively improve themselves and grow. An order where people study and achieve degrees in the disciplines required to become an extremely good person.

I believe that humanity is supposed to be the highest order of life; however, we don't come close to being the highest order of life. People are uninspired, unintelligent, untalented, physically weak and they don't work hard, yet they couldn't be more arrogant, they even speak down of others.

Most people seem to have never stopped and taken a good hard look at themselves. They just dawdle through life and think they're awesome for no reason. Who can talk down about another person? Why does anybody think that they can speak down about anybody else? Only a person that is actively attempting and succeeding in achieving excellence may talk down about others, except for those actively pursuing excellence.

I think what the world needs, for goodness' sake, is a system of education where people can study and achieve degrees. I'm going to instigate just such a system. There will be 37 degrees that a person can earn.

The disciplines believed to be most essential to the development and growth of individuals into extremely well rounded and good people that one can study and earn degrees in are, in no particular order:

- Nutrition

- Physical Fitness and Health

- Mental Fitness and Health

- Communication Skills

- Manners and Common Sense Etiquette

- Biomechanics

- Music Appreciation

- Music Performance and Participation

- Music Theory

- Writing Skills

- Business Skills & Business Communications

- Leadership Skills

- Computer literacy

- Software Literacy

- Teaching Skills

- Know a Trade - Other than your chosen vocation and other than cooking skills.

- Media Studies

- History

- Psychology

- Objectivity

- Physics

- Mathematics

- Biology

- Micro biology

- Electronics

- Mechanics levels 1&2

- Horticulture

- Cooking Skills

- Sport Appreciation

- Sport Participation

- Dance Appreciation

- Dance Participation

- Academic Achievements Level 1 - Secondary / High School Certificate

- Academic Achievement Level 2 - Tertiary or Apprenticeship, etc.

- Driving skills and Attitude

  and

- The Order Itself

Then a man may judge another man according to the number of degrees that he has. One may also learn their place according to the number of degrees they have.

This system will require a governing body, a governing body where nobody gets paid, ever. People will be required to volunteer their time to the cause for goodness' sake.

To achieve a degree, a person will have to apply to the governing body for a portion of the examination paper so that they can have an idea of what to be studying. A person will then study on their own time and at their own expense. They will then have to apply for a complete exam paper. The exam paper will be completed and returned to the governing body for assessment, should the examination results be deemed satisfactory, a degree will be issued to the applicant at their expense, probably. This is only an idea, I think it would be great if I could make this a reality, it will require many hands and much time. If you're thinking of wanting to do something good, even intelligent, why not try to get something started in your area, for goodness' sake.

It would be absolutely brilliant if it was possible to reward people who have achieved a degree at no expense to them; however, this is the real world and everything costs money. If this governing body was to purchase certificates in acknowledgement of a person's achievements and endeavors, they would have to purchase them. This body would probably be able to get a good price if they were expecting to be able to achieve much more business for the certificate suppliers; but, it would still cost money.

Perhaps it will work if people want to invest the small amounts to receive a physical certificate to acknowledge their achievement if it came down to investing in their personal development; however, I think that this is easily said by somebody from a middle class family from a city in Australia. There must be way. A way for people to be able to study and achieve degrees in certain disciplines and be rewarded with a physical certificate, a nice one, and something to acknowledge that they have achieved enough degrees to reach a certain level.

People will have to be able to prove that they have done this work and that they really have achieved the degrees that they claim to have achieved. Certificates is the logical answer; but, they don't travel very well. People are going to want to have something that they can either wear or keep in their pocket, purse or wallet. This will have to be something that cannot be replicated cheaply and easily. This will cost money also. The expenses involved will include certificates and an acknowledgement of one's level that one will be able to carry on their person.

Nobody gets paid. Nobody is to make any money, at all, in this pursuit of goodness. One must volunteer their time to organise something in their communities if they so desire. The only cost to anybody is what was previously stated, there might be some small mailing expenses as well. No governing body is to make any money, no person is to take donations or be remunerated in any way if they do decide they would like to help me in my endeavor. I don't want to be a complete tightwad; however, I am quite a bit of a tightwad and I do get quite serious sometimes. It would be great if people would help me and there should be many benefits to helping me with this by starting up something in your community. Any work a person does towards this is something they will be able to add to their Curriculum Vitae and will help them to achieve professional development and growth.

All anybody would really need is a computer with internet access. Somebody could use social networking media to create communities where they can then communicate these ideas.

People, welcome to my resolve to initiate and establish "The Order of Goodness"; however, the name might already be taken and I'm also beginning to suspect that it might suck. I think I need to think about SEO for this.

The expression, "Keep it simple stupid" (Unknown) is a fine motif that constantly inspires me to, well, keep it simple and to make sure I'm doing the little things correctly, the little things that make up the larger things. It's imperative that I make sure I'm not trying to reinvent the wheel.

Now, honestly, get out there and start building a community. Unite people by communication, communication about "The Order of Goodness", for goodness' sake.

Positivity begets positivity, negativity begets negativity. Positive actions, positive reactions; negative actions, negative reactions.

This is the essential principle of Karma. Karma is physically real; however, it isn't a mystical force, it is a matter of probability. I'm not sure if I mentioned it earlier in the piece; but, I don't believe in accidents. I even believe that most, if not all, accidents are so avoidable that you could even work them happening out on paper before they happen.

If you're not doing anything wrong, you're not going to get caught doing something wrong and you won't have to face the consequences. If you're not being a knob, people aren't going to want to tell anybody you're a knob. It's Karma and Karma is very easy to understand. Karma is also physically real and exists on planet earth. This is proven beyond any reasonable doubt.

If you're not being a knob, nobody will want to tell anybody that you're a knob, unless they are gigantic knobs themselves, which is what unfortunately happened to me. Because such pathetic accusations where so far out of character for me, it became increasingly clear just what gigantic knobs the people accusing me of these things were. Why would they bother? Why wouldn't anybody ask me about what they were hearing about me? I eventually worked myself out of it and the psychopaths with nothing better to do than rat on me and get me in trouble for things I would never think to do in the first place and something that required X-ray vision to be doing have to face the consequences now. Psychopaths with no intelligence or talent to think of something better to do. They were found out in the end and now they have to face the consequences while I'm still working on getting out of this, damned pieces of rodent excrement.

Just think about it, not that I am accusing anybody of having to be told this, if you pass a stranger on a street what will happen if you smile at him or her? They'll probably smile back.

What else? They will probably continue smiling, then others will see them smiling, they might smile at everyone they pass, they will probably smile back and be much happier for it as well, and so on and so on. A positive spiral.

What will happen if you pass a stranger on the street and you attack or threaten them or even physically attack them unprovoked? Use your imagination. Don't only think of the immediate reaction, there will also be further negative reactions. How long will it take for the stories of people that have been attacked unprovoked and your name to come together? Then what? HUH??

Karma is physically real and it exists on planet earth. Karma is not a mystical force with a consciousness. Karma is a matter of probability. Keep your actions, thoughts and words positive and you can't get into much trouble. Do you want to stay out of trouble, because who could be bothered with trouble? Then keep this in mind at all times.

I can't believe I haven't even written anything about this next bit either. I guess it just didn't come up. What is it? It is physically real and exists on planet earth. It is a part of everybody's day, every day? It is the epitome of badness and evil?

It is the Devil.

It's real man. It's around you every day. You see it every day. You see it every day; but, you don't know what it is. The Devil exists on planet earth; it always has and always will. "The Devil" is anything that tempts you to do something you know is wrong. The Devil is the temptation itself. It could be a friend, a family member, a boss or co-worker. It could simply be inside you. It should be one's mission to always resist and remain above the temptation to do something that they know is wrong.

The Devil is real.

It exists and is all around us, everyday. It is even inside us, in our heads.

"Every single one of us has the devil inside" (INXS, 1987).

You have to be strong and do the right thing, every time. The Devil will always exist and we simply must not allow ourselves to be too weak to maintain resistance.

I actively decided that I wanted to be an upstanding, law abiding, contributing and valuable member of society. I got in trouble when I was growing up and quickly learnt that I couldn't be bothered with being in trouble, I wanted to try to be funny instead, I wanted to be loved, I wanted to have the best attitude a person could have, I wanted to play music, I wanted to play drums, I wanted to get a good job, I wanted to buy a good house, I wanted to buy several more. I didn't have time to get in trouble and any trouble I did get in would really hurt my chances of being able to accomplish these things. I wanted to never set a foot wrong.

While I was actively always doing the right thing, I noticed that it either costs more money or there was significantly more work involved to do the right thing. I love putting in, I love doing all of that extra work. The work that I put in to do the right thing every time makes me feel better.

Do you always do the right thing? Think about it. Take a good hard look at yourselves and the world around you.

Littering, including littering cigarette butts, speeding, gossiping, lying, backstabbing, name calling, talking on a mobile phone while driving, illegal downloading of licensed digital material, not listening, surely I've hit something that you do commonly. It's wrong; but, you still do it and probably often. You might not even realise you're doing it. Why do you do it anyway? Temptation.

Temptation to do the wrong thing because doing the right thing costs more money and is more work.

Always doing the right thing is hard. It is a lot of work. People act up and misbehave because it is easy. It's simply succumbing to the temptation and it is very easy. Being right on top of your game and always having excellent manners, an excellent attitude, performing excellently at your job and actively doing the right thing every time is hard, very hard. That's why nobody just does the right thing every time.

The people that always do the right thing are the truly strong. The people who act up and misbehave are the weak who easily give in to temptation, weak people that cannot resist the devil.

I don't see any reason to worry about a red goat legged fellow with a pitchfork, pointy tail, horns and a goatee beard coming to steal your soul and taking it to hell or anything. I think that's the bogey man, and only children believe in the bogey man.

In the story of Adam and Eve in the Garden of Eden, A fictitious deity character specifically tells Eve not to eat the fruit from a tree. Eve then knew that doing so was wrong. Temptation came and began to lure Eve into doing it anyway. Eve wasn't able to resist the temptation, the devil. Then, because Eve wasn't able to resist the temptation she was evicted from the garden, from paradise. Adam was also evicted from the garden for Eve's misbehavior, disobedience and weakness.

This is not a documentary of history, to see it as such is to fool oneself and is also the product of literary works being misconstrued. The actual meaning of the story was this; Adam and Eve are representative of all people, this really means YOU. If ANYBODY cannot resist the temptation to do something they know is wrong and have specifically been told is wrong, then NOBODY gets to live in paradise. The garden of Eden is representative of what the world, on planet earth, would be like today, right now, if everybody had the strength to resist the temptation, to resist the devil. If everybody had the strength to resist the devil every time we would all live in paradise, a place with no pain. Here, now. In this life. This one life. The only life you will ever know.

Every decision a person makes every day affects the entire world. It may be difficult to see yourself as being able to influence the entire world; but, every decision you make every day affects the entire world. Choose to be your best all the time; choose to have the strength to resist the devil all the time. Only when every person can resist the devil every time can we live in paradise.

That said, or written, you're allowed to make mistakes. Making mistakes is part of being human, it's going to happen, you are going to make mistakes. Don't stress, it's not like the devil then owns you for one million years or anything, you're going to make mistakes. The idea is that you make mistakes and then you learn from them and grow, then you become a better person. Smart people do stupid things, they just don't do the same stupid thing twice, well, they definitely don't do the same stupid thing three times. You're allowed to make mistakes, you're simply going to make mistakes, you're not necessarily doing anything wrong or being bad.

I'm a Jazz musician. I studied Jazz for years to learn that there was nothing to know about Jazz, nothing at all. Learning what an "AABA structure" is and how to play "triplets" will help; but, there is nothing to know about Jazz. Jazz is the product of making mistakes. If people didn't make mistakes Jazz music wouldn't exist. Screw that, I love Jazz. That means that making mistakes is a good thing.

Good things happen and people learn when mistakes are made. There's no doubt that you've learnt from other people's mistakes as well as your own. Jazz came from people playing popular songs of the time and making mistakes as they did so. They made the observation that it sounded cool when they made mistakes. If they made a mistake they could play something else to cover it up or make it right. This sounded cool and made the songs different. The story ends with improvisation. These people then decided to make mistakes deliberately, this is how Jazz happened. I'm so glad it did. I love playing Jazz because you can do anything you feel like, you try to make it nice; but, you get to go as big as you feel like as well, it's great, it's fun.

To bring around the point again, you're going to make mistakes and when you do there's no need to panic. What matters most is what you play next. When you make a mistake it is what you do next that either corrects the situation or compounds your folly. In more simple English, it's what you do next that either makes it right or makes it worse. When you make a mistake, don't run away or deny it, don't try to justify it, don't get offended and think you're above making mistakes, just accept it. You're going to make mistakes, I've made mistakes. When you make a mistake you should just say to yourself, I've made a mistake, I'm not above making mistakes, everybody makes mistakes and what matters most is what I play next. Accept it, admit it, learn from it, develop and grow. Then who are you going to annoy? Who's going to want to wish you harm then?

Another thing that I think is worth communicating to you is that you're going to make mistakes and your first mistake could be a kill. You have to know your place and know what's going on around you. You have to be serious some times.

I don't think I have any more to write and that this is the end of the book.

Thanks for coming; this was my book of what I've learnt, containing most of what I've learnt and a few extra bits for flavouring. I hope you will continue the direction you have already chosen to take by reading this book and continue to want to be absolutely awesome. That means, want to be absolutely awesome and not just decide for yourself that you're absolutely awesome; but, you don't really do anything and probably don't even do a very good job at what you do do. There's a big difference. Know the difference, experience the difference. Now get on the floor and do twelve push ups. Do this as often as possible. Push. Push yourself, push the boundaries, push the limits.

To finish off, I only have a few more things to add. The first is that a degree with The Order of Goodness will not be regarded as equivalent to an academic degree. It is planned that a degree will require only a few months of study to achieve and any curriculum is currently in the works, this doesn't mean that you can't still be proactive about building or joining an order of goodness community while it is still in its development stage. Every step is a step in the right direction.

Furthermore, one is expected to only participate in or commit to the order of goodness on a part time basis. Everybody is encouraged to be developing their professional lives, have a full time job or be studying full time towards achieving a full time job.

Any participation in the order is to be considered a supplement to one's professional development.

Moreover, rubbish goes in a rubbish bin, rubbish goes in a rubbish bin, rubbish goes in a rubbish bin, rubbish goes in a rubbish bin and rubbish goes in a rubbish bin. A rubbish bin is the place for rubbish, rubbish's place is in a rubbish bin. A place for everything and everything in its place. When things aren't in their places accidents happen. I don't believe in accidents, I only believe in ignorance, stupidity and negligence. Rubbish needs to be in its place too. Littering is abhorrent, this includes littering of cigarette butts, they go in a bin or an ashtray and nowhere else. Every time you put a cigarette butt or any other piece of garbage anywhere other than in a rubbish bin where it belongs you are doing the wrong thing. You are succumbing to the temptation of the devil like a weak pathetic little bitch.

Now, be good, please. Always do the right thing just because you can.

"As long as you're learning, you're growing" (Me, 2013)

• www.blakejoy.com

Oh, I might also add that I kept changing my bands' names and realised that I couldn't keep updating my them in my book, so I"ll keep a space for my music projects at www.blakejoy.com so people can keep up to date with the names of my various musical projects. Honestly, if you want good music from a guy that really puts in to make his music good and worth listening to keep an eye out at blakejoy.com, please.

"Cheers Big Ears!" (Unknown).

\*\*\*\*

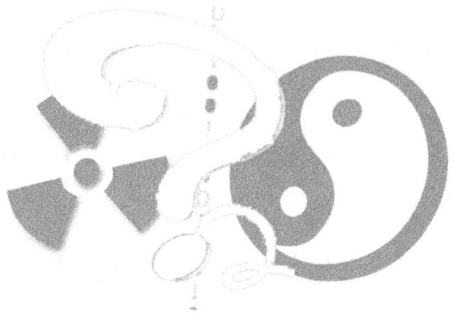

## The Bit Before the First Bit that I Wrote Last and Also Comes Last Now.

I Wrote this part of the book after I had finished the main body. I originally placed it at the beginning of the book so there is all this stuff about being the beginning of the book. I just decided that for this edition I would place these parts at the end of the book instead and begin this edition with the actual first chapter. Instead of editing it so that it doesn't read like the beginning I'm going to leave it, please enjoy!

This is the bit that comes at the start of the book. I think they usually call it a "Pre-word" or "Preface" or "Introduction". I explain who I am and why I'm doing this in the first chapter so there's no need to explain any of this here. I think I might use this as a place to put all the disclaimers to inform readers of things they might need to be aware of when approaching this book. I kept it pretty tame; but, I have to be honest and objective. There were a few

"F-words" later on so I have had to edit the whole book to either not include any profanity or to soften the blow a little. It isn't anywhere near as funny as it was, it wasn't very funny in the first place; but, now it's even less funny than that. Ah well. I recommend that you also buy the other one with the restricted rating.

Please don't read any further if you're a little bit sensitive and don't take kindly to be spoken down to, you big baby. You have to be tough and accept negative criticism. Maynard from the band "Tool" said to me, indirectly, that, "You have to be your own worst critic". I've held onto this saying ever since. It is important to be your own worst critic; but, who is? In my experience I've observed that most people are stupid and absolutely insane; however, they couldn't be more full of themselves. This has to be a big problem for the world. Do your bit to not become like this or knock it off if you are. What's the point of everybody thinking they're awesome and already know it all, especially teenagers? You never stop learning and you never stop growing, this stupid attitude has no place in a good world. You don't know it all, nobody does. If this offends you, you're wrong.

I'm going to use this opportunity to write in a few things I have only remembered now after I have finished writing the main body of this book. I forgot a few important things. The previous paragraph is one of them. Learn you place already, damn. You're not awesome, you're a plebeian, a tax payer, a tax file number, a commuter; shut up! Stupid bloody kids! "Destroy your ego, trust your brain" is a quote from Danny Carey, also of the band "Tool", that has become quite significant to my development. I never can understand what any of these people think they have to be so arrogant about. Good, worthwhile people don't have the time to imagine such false impressions of themselves, it seems.

So what are a few important things I should probably put in this book but haven't yet? Don't stand or sit around waiting for the clock when you're at work, you're stuck there, put in. The reason I have always kept as busy as possible while I'm at work is simply because I don't want to be at work and be on somebody else's time. I kept myself nice and busy so I didn't have to think about it. That way, the time seems to go so much faster. I kept myself busy and the next thing I knew I was on my own time again; I also had money in the bank.

This is one of those times that you're going to have to toughen up and not be easily offended, cry-baby. I'm using this introduction piece as a place to put some things I didn't write while I was writing the book, important things. Some of the things in this book are more important than others and this one is very important. There's a difference between goodness and trying to kiss god's arse, one's good because it's goodness. Religious authorities are each a business like any other.

If one's body doesn't transcend into the afterlife, does that mean that one's central nervous system also doesn't transcend into the afterlife? How good could heaven be if one has no eyes to see, no nose to smell, no hands to touch, no tongue to taste and no ears to hear? How bad could hell be? All anybody ever *knew* and all anybody has ever seen is one life and planet earth. You'll never know another life, whether there is another life or not. The ideas of heaven and hell reek of being made up to scare people into behaving; but, it seems to have scared them completely insane instead, scared them homicidal. Egad man.

Religious authorities aren't interested in you, your life, your happiness or what happens to you in this life or any other. They are each a business. It is their business to make you believe and scare you into believing that you need them. People of religious authorities may be very nice to you; but, think about it, of course they are, if you were running a business you would also be very nice to your customers. If you aren't nice to your customers they're going to tell people that you weren't nice to them. If you walk into a shop, the shop attendant isn't going to tell you to go away. A shop is a business and they're in business to make money and they're not going to make any money if they're rude to their customers or potential customers.

If you were evil, you wouldn't know it, you'd probably think you were doing the right thing. If you were insane you wouldn't know it either. I think what religious authorities do is make things up, scare people into believing them and then sell them the answer; which is also made up. A religious authority isn't going to tell you that there's every chance that they might be ill-informed so you can make an objective decision and approach your life based on what you *know* about the world. A religious authority will never tell you that they have no evidence because they might have been misled, misconstrued texts, or even been lied to. It isn't their business to.

There has never been any shortage of mundane reasons for a person to be on their best behavior at all times.

I think that concludes this preface. Please hang in there and keep reading. You might want to have a book mark handy too. I deliberately started writing this book with no form or structure at all. I figured that everything is relevant to one time and one place, being planet earth and now, or the last few millennia and it should all come together and make sense in the end; however, I could be wrong, in which case, meh! I just hope it's an interesting experience then. This book is pretty much entirely ad-libbed with some additions and editing at the end. The chapters might get quite long, even painful, so have a book mark handy. I just threw in a break and a change of topic every so often. Just keep reading, you'll get to the end then realise you have forgotten everything but the last few pages anyway. You might need to read this through several times to get the full experience.

Anyway, I'm not doing this preface anymore. So, to wrap it up, stop thinking you're absolutely awesome for no reason, if you were really that good, other people would be saying it for you, shut up, do your work, do a good job and let other people do the talking for you, damn man.

In other words, please enjoy my book titled "What I've learnt and what I was thinking behind their backs". I'm sorry I couldn't make it funnier.

Now, for the feature presentation...please enjoy, or something.

****

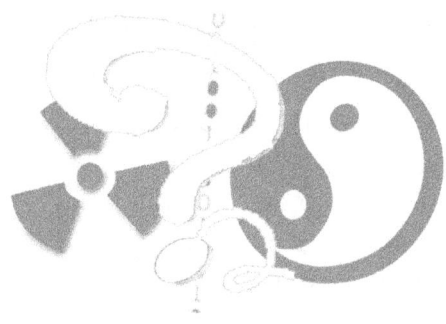

## The Second Bit Before the First Bit That I Wrote Last and Also Comes Last Now.

I know I said (or whatever) it was time for the feature presentation; but, I was mistaken. Now I'm going to start a whole new section that will go before the main body of this book. Well, it did go before the main part; however, I wrote it after the main body and it comes after the main body now. K?

A few more things that I have failed to communicate thus far in this book, because I'm writing this bit last, are:

The bit about how there is an underlying pattern to life and to nature. The underlying pattern to life is:

Being born, being raised, getting educated, getting a job, finding a mate, buying a house, reproducing, raising them until they grow up into fine individuals and then watching them do the same thing. You might even get the chance to watch your children's children's children grow up, find a mate, reproduce and then raise a fine person in your lifetime. That's what it's all about. There's no need to be belligerent or obnoxious, just get into life. Get out there and do the natural thing. Get an education, get some experience, get a job, find a friend, buy a house, have a kid or two, raise them into fine pillars of the community and then watch them do the same thing.

Also, if you're driving along and a motorist is indicating that they wish to change lanes because they probably need to. Do you:

Back off the accelerator a little and allow them to merge into the lane you are in ahead of you like a sane person?

or

Do anything other than back off the accelerator a little and allow them to merge into the lane you are in ahead of you like a sane person?

This is more like a rant than an exceptionally important communication. There is merit to everything you have or will read in this book. It might just take some thinking about, and being objective about, before you can fully appreciate it.

What would a person have to have wrong with them to see a person indicating that they wish to change lanes and simply not allow them to? I've seen this a few times while I have been on the roads and I have also had a lunatic refuse to allow me to merge into a lane ahead of her. What is wrong with some people?

What's wrong with being nice and considerate and thoughtful of other motorists, et cetera, and their needs? What's wrong with being friendly and kind? What's wrong with doing the *right* thing because you can?

I have a few more things to touch on that I probably could have touched on in the main body of this book; but, the story didn't lead there and I missed them. I'm going to write them in now because I don't think they'll fit into the stories if they didn't go there the first time. Who cares anyway? This book deliberately has no form or organisation, I hope it's fun as well as mind blowing-ly educational and enlightening. I think you might have to read this book over a few times to get the most of it. I hope it makes a good reference tool as well.

Everything had to come from somewhere, you know?

The laws of physics only work one way, you know?

The laws of physics only work one way and they are the same for everybody. Who do you like the most? If anybody else can do something you can too, well, almost anything. Height and weight become variables in the equation; but, if you admire or idolise somebody you can do just about anything they can do. It's just a matter of practicing and understanding the laws of physics and the laws of nature and how they affect your body.

What's the difference between you and a person you admire for their athletic prowess for example? You might have a different height or weight and that might affect how the forces of nature impede or work against your bodies when it comes to performing.

Everything had to come from somewhere. EVERYTHING!!!

Everything of this earth can be traced back from where it came, meaning everything that *is* of this earth.

Another thing I should add is that I'm Australian. Yeah Yeah, I'm embarrassed by the accents too! I can't do much about it. It's just an unfortunate part of life that I have to be born with one of these hideous accents. I don't know how relevant this will be as I'm not sure I'll even sell any of these in Australia, let alone, overseas; but, who knows? In these days of the digital media it's probably quite likely that I might sell a few abroad. The point of this is that in Australia we spell a few things differently, like, "Arse", and we drive on the left side of the road. For countries other than Australia, that drive on the incorrect side of the road, you have to change all the left to right and so forth.

There's no good in driving on the left, and keeping left, if you're supposed to be on the right hand side, that would make you a maniac man, I don't recommend it.

Also, if a parked or stationary car is in your lane on a two lane road, it is your responsibility to give way to traffic coming the other way that does not have a vehicle obstructing its lane. Not giving way to traffic coming towards you when you have a vehicle blocking your lane is also called "driving into oncoming traffic" and it is absolutely retarded. I can't believe I even see these things on the road and that I would actually make a mental note to include them in this book.

People couldn't be more ignorant. I'm honestly not trying to offend anybody or trying to pick a fight with anybody, especially customers, I'm really just being honest. Please just accept it as being an objective observation. Nobody is infallible and perfection does not exist. Everybody makes mistakes and everybody will make mistakes. I'm not interested in fighting or offending people, I just have to be honest and present my observations in an honest and objective manner. There are many problems with society and with many individuals, there's absolutely no good in not being able to accept that you can make mistakes. You can't help making mistakes and it really is embarrassing when somebody is too weak to accept they have made a mistake. An understanding and peaceful global community cannot exist as long as any people are too arrogant or stupid and think they know it all, or if people are too weak to accept they can make, or have made, a mistake. That's asking for trouble.

Also, as well as having horrible accents, in Australia we also use an "S" when we spell words that end in "ise" or "ize" instead of a "Z", which is essential to know, just like EVERYTHING HAD TO COME FROM SOMEWHERE!

Cool, I think it's time to get to the actual beginning of this book now. I hope you enjoy this and I hope many people learn and are inspired or enlightened by my, and a few other's, observations that I think are important to communicate to a new, hopefully broader, audience.

I haven't mentioned anything about "How to Operate Your Brain" by Dr. Timothy Leary yet either (1994). I think I'm going to end the introductory part of this book with a passage from, "How to Operate Your Brain" as I think it is a fine piece of journalism and should definitely be included in and communicated to a new, broader, audience. Like "Tool" before me. Actually I think I'm going to end the entire book with this now! Sweet! Bonzer! F.N-YEAH!!!

So now, for the last time before I stop remembering things that I should have put in this book but didn't and let you get to the actual first chapter and proper beginning of this book, or actually the ending now, I will transcribe, for your reading pleasure, or experience, a passage from, "How to Operate Your Brain", by Dr. Timothy Leary, please enjoy!

How to Operate Your Brain.

Think for Yourself, Question Authority.

Think for Yourself, Question Authority.

Throughout human history as our species has faced the frightening, terrorising fact that we do not know who we are or where we are going in this ocean of chaos, it is then the authorities, the political, the religious, the educational authorities that attempted to comfort us by giving us order, rules and regulations, informing, forming in our minds, their view of reality.

To think for yourself you must question authority and learn how to put yourself in a state of vulnerable open-mindedness, chaotic confused vulnerability, to inform yourself.

Think for Yourself, Question Authority

Think for Yourself, Question Authority.

# REFERENCES

**Anselmo, Phil.** *"Is there no standard anymore?"*and *"Be yourself by yourself, stay away from me, a lesson learnt in life, known from the dawn of time, RE-SPECT"* from the song "Walk", Pantera, from the album "Vulgar Display of Power", 1992, Atco/East West and Rhino Records.

*"There's a lot to learn from a bottle of whiskey"*, from the song "Where you Come From", Pantera, from the album "Official Live: 101 Proof", 1997, East West.

**Beastie Boys.** *"Come on y'all it's time to get nice"*, from the song "Brass Monkey", from the album "Licensed to Ill", 1986, Def Jam/Columbia.

*"Open up your ears and clean out your eyes"*, from the song "Alive", appearing on the album "The Sounds of Science", 1999, Capitol Records and Grand Royal.

**Bell, Burton C.** *"All I know is what I read"*, from the song "Cyberwaste", from the album Archetype, Fear Factory, 2004, Liquid 8.

**Bjork.** *"If you complain once more you'll meet an army of me."*, from the song "Army of me", from the album "Post", 1995, One Little Indian.

**Black Eyed Peas.** *"Where is the love?"*, from the song "Where is the Love?", Black Eyed Peas featuring Justin Timberlake, from the album "E l e p h u n k", 2 0 0 3, A & M, will.i.am, Interscope.

**Boyd, Brandon.** *"You'd better think fast because you never know what's coming around the bend"* and *"Consequence is a bigger word than you think"*, from the song "Consequence".

*"Don't let the world bring you down, not everyone here is that (messed up) and cold"* ^ and *"...leave in my wake a trail of fear"* and *"... leaving the air behind me clear"*, from the song "The Warmth". ^ Actual quote has been edited f o r    g e n e r a l exhibition. Source has a restricted rating, contains mild coarse language.

*"The man standing in front of me doesn't know why he's waiting or what he's waiting for. Maybe it's mean; but, I'm sick of wasting energy, maybe if I look in my heart I can find a back door"*, from the song "Privilege".

*"Make Yourself"* and *"If I hadn't made me, I would have been made somehow, if I hadn't assembled myself I'd have fallen apart by now"*, from the song "Make Yourself".

From the album "Make Yourself", Incubus, 1999, Immortal Records and Epic.

**Carey, Danny.** *"Destroy your ego, trust your brain".* Unknown Date. Unknown Source.

**Cavalera, Max.** *"I'm one for the rules!",* from the song "Inner Self", Sepultura, from the album "Beneath the Remains", 1989, Roadrunner.

> *"Pain makes me stronger every day"* and *"Life is chaos, you gotta deal with it",* from the song "Clenched Fist", Sepultura, from the album "Chaos AD", 1996, Roadrunner Records and Epic.

**Claypool, Les.** *"Caution should be used while driving a motor vehicle or operating machinery",* song title, Sausage, from the album "Riddles are Abound Tonight", 1994, Interscope and Prawn Song.

> *"Jerry was a race car driver, he drove so god damned fast, he never did win (no) checkered flags but he never did come in last"* and *"Jerry was a race car driver, twenty-two years old, one too many...one night, wrapped himself around a telephone pole",* from the song "Jerry was a Race Car Driver", Primus, from the album, "Sailing the Seas of Cheese", 1991, Interscope.

**Cypress Hill.** *"A to the (expletive) K homeboy, A to the (expletive)K",* from the song "A to the K", from the album "Black Sunday", 1993,

Ruffhouse and Columbia. Actual quote has been edited for general exhibition, contains strong coarse language.

**De La Rocha, Zac.** *"Know your enemy".*

*"Word is born, fight the war, (ignore) the norm".*^

*"So sick of complacence".*

*"What? The land of the free? Whoever told you that is your enemy".*

from the song "Know your Enemy", from self titled album, Rage Against the Machine, 1992, Epic. ^ Actual quote has been edited for general exhibition, contains strong coarse language.

**Dream Theatre.** *"You'll find all you need in your mind if you take the time",* from the song "Take the Time", from the album "Images and Words", 1992, Atco.

**Harper, Ben.** *"What makes me strong is to know what makes me weak",* from the song "I Want to be Ready".

*"Every moral has a story and every story has an end. Every battle has its glory and its consequence",* from the song "Glory and Consequence".

*"I met a man who had to walk with his hands, blessed with life, cursed as man; still, he walks taller than most others can"*, from the song "The Will to Live".

From the album "The Will to Live", 1997, Virgin America.

**INXS.** *"Every single one of us has the devil inside"*, from the song "The Devil Inside", from the album "Kick", 1987, WEA, Atlantic.

**Jillette, Penn.** *"Some people are nutty enough to believe in god and the devil, and hell; but, nobody's nutty enough to take the devil's side"*, appearing on "Exorcism", season five, episode five of "Penn and Teller's Bullshit", 2007, Showtime.

**Jones, Norah.** *"There's one born every minute, sucker, so keep it in your pants, sucker"*, from the song "Sucker", Peeping Tom, self titled album, 2006, Ipecac Recordings.

**Keenan, Maynard James.** *"Who am I to judge or strike you down?"*, from the song "Pushit".

*"(Curse) all you junkies and (Curse) your short memories"*, from the song "Aenima".^

From the album "Aenima", Tool, 1996, Zoo Entertainment. ^ Actual quote has been edited for general exhibition, contains strong coarse language.

*"You have to be your own worst critic"*, from radio interview on Triple J, Unknown Date.

*"Watch the weather change"*, from the song "Disposition".

*"All this pain is an illusion"*, from the songs "Parabol" and "Parabola".

From the album "Lateralus", Tool, 2001, Volcano Entertainment.

*"Why don't you watch where you're wandering? Why don't you watch where you're stumbling?"*, from the song "Swamp Song", from the album "Undertow", Tool, 1993, Zoo Entertainment.

**Lamb**. *"Life's so precious, don't let it pass you by."*, from the song "Here".

*"There's so many things that we miss in our everyday lives, we're so busy hustling, bustling chasing far away dreams, we forget the little things, like blue skies, green eyes and our babies growing, like rainbows, fresh snow and the smell of summer, we forget to live"*, from the song "Little Things".

*"Burn like a good bonfire in whatever you do"*, from the song "Bonfire".

*"We're so busy looking for a saviour, we don't see the power in ourselves"*, from the song "Here".

From the album "Fear of Fours", 1999, Mercury Records.

**Machinehead.** *"Real eyes realise real lies."*, song title, from the album "Burn my Eyes", 1994, Roadrunner Records.

**McCartney, Paul, Linda.** *"When you've got a job to do, you've got to do it well."* from the song "Live and Let Die", 1973, Apple.

**Patton, Mike.** *"It's either you or them"*, from the song "Night of the Hunter", Fantomas, from the album "The Director's Cut", 2001, Ipecac.

*"None of them knew they were robots"*, song title, Mr Bungle, from the album "California", 1999, Warner Brothers.

*"One day the wind will come up and you'll come up empty again, who'll be laughing then? You'll come up empty again, It's always funny until someone gets hurt and then it's just hilarious"*, from the song "Ricochet", Faith No More.

*"Being good gets you stuff"*, from the song "Cuckoo For Caca", Faith No More.

From the album "King for a Day, Fool for a Lifetime", 1995, Polypro K.K. and Slash.

**Regurgitator.** *"No matter what your colour, no matter what your sex, respect"*, from the song "Pop Porn", from the album "Tu-Plang", 1996, East West/Warner Music Australia, Reprise/Warner Bros. Records.

*"I don't see a point to this place; but, I'm happy to be floating in space"*, from the song "Just Another Beautiful Story", from the album "Unit", 1997, East West Records.

**Rose, Axl.** *"It's so easy when everybody's trying to please me"* and *"You get nothing for nothing, if that's what you do then turn around (,) I've got news for you"*, from the song "It's so Easy". ^

*"Welcome to the Jungle"*, song title.

*"She used to love her heroin; but, now she's underground"*, from the song "My Michelle".

*"I'm on the night train, ready to crash and burn, I'll never learn"*, from the song "Night Train".

From the album "Appetite for Destruction", Guns n' Roses, 1987, Geffen Records. ^ Actual quote edited for general exhibition, contains strong coarse language.

"You could be mine; but, you're way out of line.", from the song "You Could be Mine", Guns n' Roses, from the album, "Use Your Illusion II", 1991, Geffen Records, UZI Suicide.

**Tyler, Steven.** *"There's something wrong with the world today, there's something wrong with our eyes",* from the song "Living on the Edge", Aerosmith, from the album "Get a Grip", 1993, Geffen Records.

**28 Days.** *"Suckers come and go, you will bite and you wont know",* from the song "Sucker", from the album "Upstyledown", 2000, Sputnik Records.

## REFERENCES CONT.

**The Abyss**, James Cameron, 1989, Lightstorm Studios, Twentieth Century Fox.

**Adaptation**, Charlie Kaufman, Spike Jonze, 2002, Good Machine, Intermedia, Propaganda Films, Saturn Films, Columbia Pictures.

**Airplane (Flying High)**, Jerry Zucker, David Zucker, Jim Abrahams, 1980, Paramount Pictures.

**'Allo 'Allo**, 1982-1992, BBC1.

**Arlington Road**, Mark Wellington, Ehren Kruger, 1999, Lakeshore Entertainment, Screen Gems, Polydor Pictures.

**Army of Darkness**, Sam Ramie, Ivan Ramie, Bruce Campbell, 1992, Dino De Laurentiis Communications, Renaissance Pictures, Universal Studios.

**Austin Powers**, Mike Myers, Jay Roach, 1997, New Line Cinema.

**The Avengers,** 1961-1969, Sydney Newman, ITV/ABC/Thames.

**Beautiful People**, Jasmin Dizdar, 1999, BFI, Trimark Pictures, Channel Four Films.

**Being John Malkovich**, Charlie Kaufman, Spike Jonze, 1999, Single Cell Pictures,

Propaganda Films, Gramercy Pictures, USA Films.

**Blazing Saddles**, Mel Brooks, Michael Hertzberg, Andrew Bergman, 1974, Warner Bros.

**Body Shots,** 1999, New Line Cinema.

**Brain Games**, 2011, National Geographic.

**Brazil**, Terry Gilliam, 1985, Embassy International Pictures N.V. Universal Studios, Twentieth Century Fox.

**The Castle**, Santo Cilauro, Rob Sitch, Jane Kennedy, Tom Gleisner, Stephen Curry, 1997, Village Roadshow, Miramax Films.

**Charade**, Stanley Donen, Peter Stone, Marc Behm, 1963, Stanley Donen Productions, Universal Pictures.

**The China Syndrome**, Michael Douglas, James Bridges, Mike Gray, T.S Cook, 1979, Columbia Pictures.

**Commando,** Arnold Schwarzanegger, 1985, Silver Pictures, Twentieth Century Fox.

**Connections**, James Burke, 1978, BBC

**Contact,** Robert Zemeckis, 1997

**The Deeper Meaning of Liff,** Douglas Adams, John Lloyd, 1990, Pan Books

**Destroyed in Seconds**, 2008, Pilgrim Films and Television, Discovery Channel.

**The Devil's Advocate**, Andrew Neiderman, Jonathan Lemon, Tony Gilroy, 1997, Regency Enterprises, Warner Bros.

**Donnie Darko**, Richard Kelly, 2001, Flower Films, Pandora Cinema, Newmarket Films.

**Evolution**, Ivan Reitman, 2001, The Montecito Picture Company, DreamWorks, Columbia Pictures.

**Existenz**, David Cronenberg, 1999, Canadian Television Fund, Harold Greenberg Fund, The Movie Network, Natural Nylon, Serendipity Films, Telefilm Canada, Alliance Atlantis, Union Generale Cinematographic, Alliance Atlantis, Dimension Films.

**Family Ties**, Gary David Goldberg, 1982-1989, NBC.

**Frontline**, Santo Cilauro, Rob Sitch, Jane Kennedy, Tom Gleisner, 1994-1997, ABC TV.

**The Hero with a Thousand Faces**, Joseph Campbell, 1949, Pantheon Books.

**How it's Made**, Gabriel Hoss, 2001, Ztele, Discovery Channel Canada, Science.

**How to Operate Your Brain**, Timothy Leary, 1994, Retinalogic, Tapeworm Video Distributors.

**Industrial Revelations**, 2002-2008, Discovery.

**The Lost Boys**, Joel Schumacher, 1987, Warner Bros.

**Malcolm in The Middle**, Linwood Boomer, 2000-2006, Fox.

**The Matrix**, Andy Wachowski, Larry Wachowski, 1999, Village Roadshow, Silver Pictures, Groucho II Film Partnership.

**The Meaning of Liff**, Douglas Adams, John Lloyd, 1983, Pan Books.

**My Name is Earl,** Greg Garcia, 2005, Amigos de Garcia Productions, Twentieth Century Fox.

**Mythbusters,** 2003-present, Discovery.

**North Shore**, 1987, Universal Pictures.

**Overhaulin'**, Chip Foose, Bud W. Brutsman, 2004, TLC, Velocity, Discovery.

**Penn & Teller: Bullshit!,** 2003-2010, Showtime.

**Penn & Teller Tell a Lie**, 2011, Discovery Channel.

**The Philadelphia Experiment**, 1984, New World Pictures, Twentieth Century Fox.

**Predator**, 1987, Gordon Company, Silver Pictures, Davis Entertainment.

**Psycho**, Alfred Hitchcock, 1960, Shamley Productions, Paramount Pictures, Universal Pictures.

**Requiem for a Dream**, Darren Aronofsky, 2000, Thousand Words, Protozoa Pictures.

**Scrubs**, Bill Lawrence, 2001, NBC, ABC.

**Seconds From Disaster**, 2004, Darlow Smithson Productions, National Geographic Channel.

**Shutter Island,** Martin Scorsese, 2010, Appian Way Productions, Phoenix Pictures, Sikelia Productions, Paramount Pictures.

**The Simpsons**, Matt Groening, 1989, Fox.

**Sin City**, Robert Rodriguez, 2005, Troublemaker Studios, Dimension Films.

**So I Married an Axe Murderer**, 1993, Tristar Pictures.

**South Park**, Trey Parker, Matt Stone, 1997, Celluloid Studios, Braniff Productions, Parker-Stone Studios, Comedy Central.

**South Park, Bigger, Longer and Uncut,** Matt Stone, Trey Parker, Pam Brady, 1999, Comedy Central Films, Braniff Productions, Paramount Pictures, Warner Bros.

**The Spy who Shagged Me,** Mike Myers, 1999, Eric's Boy, Moving Pictures, Team Todd, New Line Cinema, Alliance Atlantis.

**Synecdoche, New York,** Charlie Kaufman, 2008, SKE, Sony Pictures Classics.

**Team America World Police,** Matt Stone, Trey Parker, 2004, Scott Rudin Productions, Paramount Pictures.

**Terminator 2**, James Cameron, 1991, Carioca Pictures, Lightstorm Entertainment, Pacific Western, StudioCanal.

**Test Your Brain,** 2011, National Geographic Channel.

**Who The (Bleep)...,** 2013, Investigation Discovery, Sirens Media.

**Who The (Bleep) Did I Marry?,** 2010 - Present, Investigation Discovery, Sirens Media.

**The Writer's Journey,** Christopher Vogler, 1992, Michael Wiese Productions.

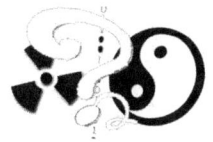

Thank you for reading!